This book is to be returned on or before
the last date stamped below.

PETTERSSON, H.

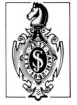

Holger Pettersson and Derek C.F. Harwood-Nash

CT and Myelography of the Spine and Cord

Techniques, Anatomy and Pathology in Children

With 93 Figures

Springer-Verlag
Berlin Heidelberg New York 1982

Holger Pettersson, MD, PhD
Clinical Assistant, Department of Radiology,
The Hospital for Sick Children, Toronto, Canada.
Assistant Professor of Radiology,
University of Lund, Sweden.

Derek C.F. Harwood-Nash, MB, ChB, FRCP(C)
Professor of Radiology,
University of Toronto, Canada.
Radiologist-in-Chief, Department of Radiology,
The Hospital for Sick Children, Toronto, Canada.

in association with
Charles R. Fitz, MD and Sylvester Chuang, MD
Division of Special Procedures,
Department of Radiology,
The Hospital for Sick Children, Toronto, Canada.

ISBN 3-540-11322-3 Springer-Verlag Berlin Heidelberg New York
ISBN 0-387-11322-3 Springer-Verlag New York Heidelberg Berlin

Library of Congress Cataloging in Publication Data
Pettersson, Holger. CT and myelography of the spine and cord. Bibliography: p. Includes index.
1. Spine — Radiography. 2. Spinal cord — Radiography. 3. Pediatric neurology — Diagnosis.
4. Tomography. 5. Myelography. 6. Pediatric radiography. I. Harwood-Nash, Derek C. II. Title.
III. Title: C.T. and myelography of the spine and cord. [DNLM: 1. Myelography — In infancy and
childhood. 2. Tomography, X-ray computed — In infancy and childhood. 3. Spine — Radiography.
4. Spinal diseases — In infancy and childhood. 5. Spinal cord diseases — In infancy and childhood.
WL 405 P499c] RJ488.5.T65P47 618.92'097560757 82-5592
ISBN 0-387-11322-3 (U.S) AACR2

Typeset by Polyglot Pte Ltd, Singapore
Printed by BAS Printers Limited, Over Wallop, Hampshire

2128/3916-543210

Preface

To study the phenomenon of disease without
books is to sail an uncharted sea. While to
study books without patients is not to go to sea
at all.

Sir William Osler

Over a period of five years, the impact of computed tomography
(CT) on pediatric neuroradiology at The Hospital for Sick Children,
Toronto, has been, as expected, in the assessment of the brain and its
abnormalities. Concurrent with this application was the introduction
of Metrizamide (Amipaque, Nyegaard & Co. AS, Oslo, Norway), a
water-soluble CSF contrast medium, used primarily as a myelographic agent. The subsequent application of the wide-aperture CT
scanner to imaging of the spine in children provided remarkable
advances in the clinical management of spinal disease since CT is far
more accurate than standard neuroradiologic procedures. The combination of CT and Metrizamide added a further dimension to the
imaging of the spine and of the spinal cord and nerve roots.

Such spinal CT and CT Metrizamide myelography in children now
occupies a significant part of day-to-day pediatric neuroradiologic
practice. They have dramatically enhanced our understanding of the
normal anatomy and pathologic entities of the spine and its contents
in children; have altered and improved the surgical management of
such diseases; and have significantly improved the clinical management of such diseases in the specialties of neurosurgery, orthopedic
surgery, and genito-urinary surgery.

This book is a complete and concise presentation of the technique
of CT Metrizamide myelography: the range of normal and abnormal
images obtained with this technique, its efficacy, and its complications. The images are now of a high resolution quality. Together with
a clinical understanding of children, they will help physicians in a
wide range of specialties, from general radiology to pediatric neurosurgery, however many children they deal with, in their understanding of this most fascinating and complicated organic system that is the
spine and its contents.

We sincerely hope that this book will provide a foundation for the
effective present and future use of this exciting technique.

Acknowledgements

We wish to express our sincere gratitude and appreciation to the following institutions and people:

Winthrop Laboratories, Aurora, Canada, and T.A. Bioteknik AB., Malmo, Sweden, for valuable financial support.

General Electric Medical Systems, Canada and the U.S.A., for their cooperation and encouragement.

The Radiologists and the previous and present Fellows of our department for advice and professional contributions.

The nursing and technical staff, in particular Anna Rusztyn, for their remarkable expertise and enthusiasm to obtain the best out of each examination.

The Neurosurgeons, Drs. Bruce Hendrick, Harold Hoffman, and Robin Humphreys, as well as the Neuropathologist, Dr. Larry Becker, for being the foundation of a truly effective clinical team.

The photographic personnel and Mary Casey, artist, in the Department of Visual Education for their patience, cooperation and skill.

The secretaries, in particular Gladys Clarke and Gail Abdool, for their efficient and conscientious work.

And last, but not least, our families for showing the understanding and patience that they have done for so long.

Contents

Abbreviations Used in the Text

MM

Metrizamide myelography. Myelography performed with conventional radiologic methods after subarachnoid administration of Metrizamide by needle puncture in the lumbar or cervical region. Plain standard radiographs and conventional tomograms of the spinal canal, cord and roots are obtained.

CTMM

Computed tomographic Metrizamide myelography. Myelography performed with computed tomography (CT) after subarachnoid administration of Metrizamide. CT sections, perpendicular to the spine or in other planes, are obtained. The examination may be a primary CTMM, in which no conventional MM is performed, or a secondary CTMM, which is a CTMM performed within the first 4 h following a conventional MM.

Chapter 1
Introduction

Its touches of beauty should never be halfway,
thereby making the reader breathless
instead of content.
The rise, the progress, the setting of imagery,
should
like the sun, come natural.

John Keats, Letters 51, 1818

Of such criteria are the standards of images, clinical understanding, technical ingenuity and diagnostic inquisitiveness made. Concomitant with artistic excellence of CT images is clinical, scientific, and diagnostic success. A step towards such goals is the application of high-resolution CT, both alone and together with a safe water-soluble CSF contrast medium.

At the Hospital for Sick Children, Toronto, as elsewhere, there has been a minor revolution in the diagnostic imaging of the spine and cord. The use of complex motion tomography as a diagnostic modality for imaging of the spine, and of oily iodinated CSF contrast and air for imaging of the spinal cord, is now historical. A 5-year experience of CT and a water-soluble iodinated CSF contrast medium, Metrizamide, has dramatically altered and enhanced the clinical and surgical understanding of spinal and spinal cord abnormalities in children of all sizes and ages.

Metrizamide was developed in response to significant complications experienced with other water-soluble CSF contrast media, containing salts of iodinated acids, associated with a resultant hypertonicity subsequent to a high iodine concentration. This high iodine concentration is necessary to provide sufficient radiographic attenuation and thus a suitable image. The iodine anion was coupled to a cation of sodium or meglumine, and the latter, being responsible for half the osmolality of the contrast medium, provided adverse physiologic effects, without increasing its radiographic attenuation.

Almén (1969) therefore proposed a non-ionic iodinated compound with considerable reduction in osmolality, being water soluble due to suitable polar functional groups, yet possessing a sufficient iodine concentration for high radiographic attenuation. Thus was Metrizamide (Amipaque, Nyegaard & Co., AS) conceived, nurtured, examined and found clinically successful (Lindgren, 1973, 1977; Post, 1980; Sackett and Strother, 1979).

The use and the safety of Metrizamide in children, once established using standard and tomographic radiography (Barry et al., 1977; Harwood-Nash and Fitz, 1979), was then combined with CT.

Our initial technical and clinical CT experience was obtained from an Ohio-Nuclear Delta 50 scanner (Harwood-Nash and Fitz, 1979, 1980; Resjö et al., 1978, 1979). During the last 2 years, however, a General Electric CT/T 8800 with a high resolution program has provided the majority of images illustrated in this book.

The normal pediatric spine differs within itself from age to age, relative to each vertebra or one section to another with greater variation than in adults (Harwood-Nash and Fitz, 1976). Examples are progressive ossification of vertebral bodies with age, change of shape, and alterations brought about by the attainment of the erect posture. The spine is a "plastic" organ, insidiously altered and externally moulded by diseases and circumstances quite different from those in adults. Bizarre congenital anomalies are common, often bereft of logical diagnostic dissection, and altered by complex neural anomalies. The diseases, albeit often unique to childhood, are clinically unpredictable, extensive, and often disturbingly insidious in presentation.

It may be said and indeed has been so (Harwood-Nash and Fitz, 1976) that a most aggressive diagnostic imaging approach must be taken in any child with even the slightest clinical and radiologic suspicion of a spinal or spinal canal abnormality. Many are surgically treatable and the preliminary effects of the disease may be devastating, even to the subsequent osseous and neural development of the spinal organ.

The technical procedures necessary for often difficult myelography in small infants, the small size of the spine, cord and roots and indeed some abnormalities themselves, demand expertise, experience and an intimate clinical knowledge of the spectrum of spinal disease at all ages. For these reasons and in the quest of diagnostic accuracy with safety, the utilization of CT with and without Metrizamide in the CSF in children evolved. It was then evaluated and ultimately found to be most effective (Harwood-Nash and Fitz, 1980; Resjö et al., 1978).

Thus initial simple standard radiographs of the spine or digital radiographs, followed by CT and Metrizamide (CTMM), are now the diagnostic methods of choice. It is still necessary to opacify the CSF in order to obtain accurate neural images. Although it will surely be possible ultimately, direct imaging of the cord and nerve roots to match the images presented in this book will rely on developments in CT technology which are still a number of years away. Violation of the sanctity of the spinal subarachnoid space is still a necessity.

The images obtained today, presented in the following chapters, should, we believe, satisfy Keats; their beauty should provide clinical contentment; their rise and progress have provided an experience that is now quite natural to those versed in the persuasions of pediatric neuroradiologic diagnostic imaging; and such imaging will not necessarily set like the sun, but inevitably change with time to other means and modalities.

References

Almén T (1969) Contrast agent design. Some aspects on the synthesis of water soluble contrast agents of low osmolality. J Theor Biol 24: 216–226

Barry JF, Harwood-Nash DC, Fitz CR, Byrd SE, Boldt DW (1977) Metrizamide in pediatric myelography. Radiology 124: 409–418

Harwood-Nash DC, Fitz CR (1976) Neuroradiology in infants and children. CV Mosby, St Louis

Harwood-Nash DC, Fitz CR (1979) Metrizamide in children. In: Sackett JF, Strother CM (eds) New techniques in myelography. Harper and Row, Hagerstown, pp 139–166

Harwood-Nash DC, Fitz CR (1980) Computed tomography and the pediatric spine: computed tomographic metrizamide myelography in children. In: Post MJD (ed) Radiographic evaluation of the spine, Masson, New York, pp 4–33

Lindgren E (ed) (1973) Metrizamide Amipaque. A non-ionic water-soluble contrast medium. Experimental and preliminary clinical investigations. Acta Radiol [Suppl] (Stockh) 335

Lindgren E (ed) (1977) Metrizamide Amipaque. The non-ionic water-soluble contrast medium. Further clinical experience in neuroradiology. Acta Radiol [Suppl] (Stockh) 355

Post MJD (1980) (ed) Radiographic evaluation of the spine. Masson, New York

Resjö IM, Harwood-Nash DC, Fitz CR, Chuang S (1978) Computed tomographic Metrizamide myelography in spinal dysraphism in infants and children. J Comput Assist Tomogr 2: 549–558

Resjö IM, Harwood-Nash DC, Fitz CR, Chuang S (1979) Normal cord in infants and children examined with computed tomographic Metrizamide myelography. Radiology 130: 691–696

Sackett JF, Strother CM (1979) (eds) New techniques in myelography. Harper and Row, Hagerstown

Chapter 2
Technique

The performance of any radiographic examination should be considered from two different aspects, namely the management of the *patient*, and the management of the *technical equipment*.

In children, the appropriate management of the patient differs with age. The infant and small child can never be intellectually motivated for the examination. At this age, tender care and as much comfort as possible by all medical, technical, and nursing personnel will make the child less anxious. With older children, a simple explanation of the approaching examination is mandatory. Gentle treatment and confident behaviour is important at all ages; from a human point of view this will make a difficult situation easier for the child, and from a technical point of view the child will be more cooperative and thus facilitate the performance both for the patient and the examiner. Each and every step must be carefully explained as it occurs.

An accurate radiologic examination also requires good technical equipment, and the appropriate management of this should be based on thorough education and experience. This is especially important in extensive and prolonged examinations with an inherent risk of complications, as for instance with the CTMM.

Sedation and Anesthesia

If primary CTMM is performed, and thus no conventional Metrizamide myelography (MM) has preceded the CT examination, general anesthesia is not necessary. Sedation is recommended up to an age of about 8 years. We use intramuscular Nembutal (Pentobarbital) in a dose of 6 mg/kg body wt. if the weight is 15 kg or less, and 5 mg/kg body wt. if the weight is more than 15 kg, to a maximum dose of 200 mg. If necessary, a supplementary dose of 2 mg/kg body wt. may be given 20 min after the initial injection. The sedation should be given at least 20 min before the procedure. There are also other sedation schedules available, as described by Anderson and Osborn (1977).

In secondary CTMM, in which conventional MM precedes the CT examination, general anesthesia for the MM should be administered to *all* children under the age of about 6, and is advisable in about 60% of children between 6 and 12 years. This general anesthesia is then continued during the CTMM. In older children, general anesthesia is seldom necessary, and then sedation as described above may be given.

Puncture of the Thecal Sac

Lumbar puncture in the prone or decubitus position should be used as the routine method. Thin 21 or 22 gauge needles are used, which decrease the likelihood of leakage of CSF and Metrizamide after the removal of the needle. Such extradural leak of Metrizamide diminishes the information obtainable at the conventional MM, although it does not interfere with the information at CTMM (see Fig. 3.11, p. 32). Also, the leak of CSF is the main cause of the headache and vomiting of the post-lumbar-puncture syndrome (Tourtellotte et al., 1972).

Low-lying lesions in the spinal canal are common in children referred for myelography. The needle puncture therefore should be directed to the lateral part of the subarachnoid space, with fluoroscopic control if necessary, to avoid direct puncture of, for instance, a low-lying conus or a tethered cord (Pettersson et al., 1982). The puncture should be performed carefully and the advancement of the needle should be stopped as soon as the "dural click" is felt. The risk for local damage caused by lumbar puncture and contrast medium injection is diminished with this technique (see Chap. 10). Cervical puncture using the lateral route at the level C1–C2 as described by Amundsen (1977) is seldom necessary, but may be used to assess the spinal canal craniad to a block to Metrizamide inserted initially in the lumbar area.

Metrizamide Injection

When clear CSF is obtained, a specimen of 0.5–2 ml is taken for routine analysis of sugar, protein, and electrolytes. If clinically indicated, or if the CSF is not clear, supplementary specimens for cytology and bacterial culture may also be obtained. Metrizamide is then slowly injected into the subarachnoid space under fluoroscopic control. If a conventional MM is first to be performed, the table should be tilted at least 20° (head up) during the injection. As the Metrizamide has a higher specific gravity than the CSF, the contrast medium will then settle in the caudal portion of the thecal sac, and this bolus of highly concentrated Metrizamide may be *carefully* manipulated to the area of interest in the spinal canal. If primary CTMM is planned, the contrast medium should be mixed as much as possible with the CSF before the examination and in these cases there is no need for upward tilting of the table.

In primary CTMM small doses of Metrizamide are used, 2 ml in the infant, and up to 7 ml in the older child, at a concentration of 170 mg iodine/ml, which is isotonic with the CSF. The patient is then tilted and rolled to mix the Metrizamide in the spinal subarachnoid space, and thence is the CT examination performed. The above-mentioned concentration of the iodine is optimal for visualization of all the dural contents in most modern CT machines. Too-large amounts of Metrizamide will create a pronounced over-range in the image, obliterating fine details and even small structures, e.g. the filum terminale.

In secondary CTMM the dose of Metrizamide given is that of the previously performed conventional MM, in which 2–12 ml Metrizamide, with a concentration varying between 170 and 250 mg iodine/ml, may be used (Fitz et al., 1977;

Sortland and Hovind, 1977). The choice of concentration should be based on the clinical history and expected findings, as well as the level of the area to be examined. The total amount given may be controlled by fluoroscopy during the Metrizamide injection. As its adverse reactions are caused by effects on the CNS, the proper maximum amount given should be related not to the weight or size of the patient, but rather to the age, as the size of the CNS is a function of age (Pettersson et al., 1982).

The Metrizamide follows the CSF circulation and is absorbed mainly intracranially. Thus the concentration of the Metrizamide–CSF solution in the spinal canal decreases with time, and the iodine concentration suitable for the secondary CTMM is obtained during the first 4 h after the Metrizamide injection.

Positioning of the Patient for CT

Neonates and small infants should be bundled in a soft towel, which will both protect them and maintain some warmth. A rubber blanket with rubber tubes containing warm running water is wrapped around the towel, as described by Harwood-Nash and Fitz (1980). Restraining bands are then placed across the wrapping to stabilize the child on the table. This wrapping is adequate to maintain normal body temperature and it will not disturb the CT image (Harwood-Nash and Fitz, 1980).

Older children are secured in a soft blanket to make them feel more comfortable, which will assist in maintaining minimal movement. The supine position is preferred, as it is the most comfortable and as the chest and abdominal movements of breathing in the prone position cause pronounced movement of the spine. The CT room should be at the ambient hospital temperature.

Observation of the Patient

If the examination is performed under general anesthesia, the child will be continuously observed by the anesthesiologist. If the patient is awake, it is often wise to have a parent or another person that the child is familiar with in the CT room. This will make the patient less anxious and thus diminish disturbing movements. The scanning area and the patient should also be observed continuously by the technician doing the examination, which is best performed via a TV camera in the CT room and a monitor at the operator console (Fig. 2.1).

Intravenous Contrast Medium Injection

Intravenous contrast medium injection may be of value in the examination of certain spinal and neural abnormalities, e.g. arteriovenous malformations or

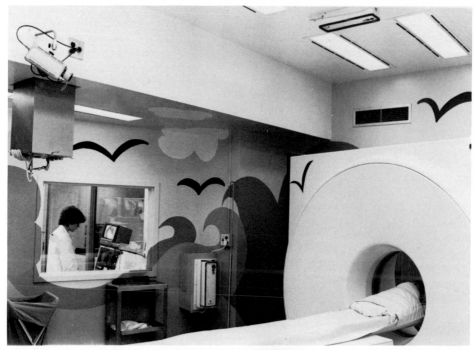

a

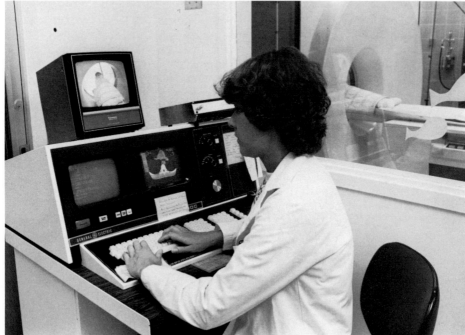

b

Fig. 2.1. CT room and operator console. The patient may be observed through the window between the operator console and CT room (a), or better via a TV camera in CT room connected to a monitor at the operator console (b). Note the wrapping of the patient.

neoplasms. In these cases we use Hypaque 60%, 3 ml/kg body wt., and most often CT sections are performed both before and immediately after the contrast medium injection.

Computed Tomographic Technique

Localization of the CT Section

1. Conventional radiograph with radiopaque ruler

Exact identification of the anatomic level of the CT section is essential. In older CT machines this may be done with a simple device that was described by Resjö et al. (1979). According to this method a plain radiograph of the spine is taken with a ruler lying underneath the patient alongside the spine. This ruler is measured at 1–cm intervals with radiopaque markers, and is attached to a 90° angled head support, applied to the vertex of the head. The head is positioned with the orbitomeatal line perpendicular to the horizontal. The patient is then placed on the scanner table in the same position as when the radiograph was taken, the ruler now being placed alongside the body, with the same relation to the vertex of the head. The levels of the scan sections are identified at the plain radiograph, and transferred to the patient's body using the ruler.

2. Digital radiograph ("Scout view")

It is now possible to obtain a digital radiograph (Scout view image—General Electric Medical Systems) of the body with modern CT equipment. As the same tube and detector system is used for the Scout view image as for the transaxial CT images, the Scout view acts as a perfect localization system (Blumenfeld, 1980). It provides excellent contrast discrimination and allows the data to be presented with different window settings. Although it does not provide as high spatial resolution as a conventional radiograph, it gives sufficient information to identify the anatomic areas to be scanned, and it also provides gross anatomic information on the lesion to be examined (Fig. 2.2).

Each section for CT scanning may be marked on the Scout view image by computed superimposition of a cursor line (Fig. 2.3).

When standard transaxial CT is performed, it is important to obtain sections as perpendicular as possible to each part of the spine, in order to assess the true size and form of the cord. To achieve this, the gantry may be angled, although this angling may be insufficient to overcome, for instance, the lower lumbar lordosis, or a severe kyphosis. In any case, the cursor line on the Scout view image reveals the true angle between the CT sections and the spine (Fig. 2.4).

It is obvious that Scout view images with cursor lines indicating the CT sections are also valuable for subsequent therapeutic intervention, e.g., surgery or therapeutic radiation.

Exposure Data and Radiation Dose

When performing conventional transaxial sections, a small scanning circle is advisable in most machines in order to obtain a large and detailed image without

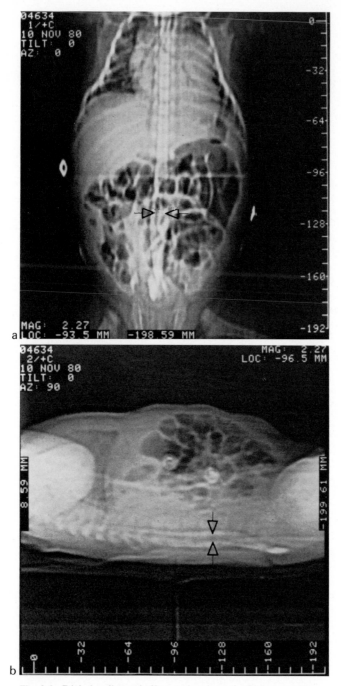

Fig. 2.2. Digital radiograph (Scout view image). Girl, 1 month.
(a) AP. The anatomic landmarks of the body are well visualized. Metrizamide in the thecal sac outlines the low cord (*arrows*), as well as the meningocele in the sacral region.
(b) Same patient, lateral Scout view. The low cord (*arrows*) is better seen than in (a) as there is no overlying bowel gas.

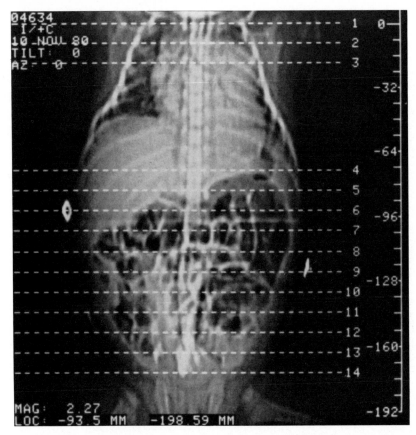

Fig. 2.3. Digital radiograph—cursor lines. Same patient as in Fig. 2.1. Cursor lines annotating the level of the CT sections are superimposed on the Scout view image.

unnecessary electronic magnification. However, if the high resolution technique described below is to be used, the largest circle should be chosen. For most purposes the thickness of the sections should be 10 mm, but in small defined areas of interest a thickness of 5 mm or 1.5 mm may be used. With the General Electric CT/T 8800 scanner we obtain images with excellent resolution using a scanning time of 9.6 s, with an exposure of 120 kV and about 120 mA. This provides a radiation dose of about 1 R (peak dose). The thinner sections demand higher doses to maintain the spatial resolution—for 5-mm cuts about 300 mA (2.5 R), and for 1.5-mm cuts about 600 mA (4.5 R).

However, we have recently used considerably lower doses, and with the "ReView" (General Electric Medical Systems) program for high resolution described below, we have obtained images of bone and Metrizamide with high spatial resolution and acceptable electronic noise. Thus exposures as small as 23 mA (about 150 mR) still give good anatomic detail (Fig. 2.5). The Scout view procedure means only a small extra dose load, averaging 75 mR.

Compared with these radiation doses, those from conventional MM are high. Rohrer et al. (1964) found that the dose for an average myelography was 800 mR — 4 R to the ovaries and 1–5 R to the third lumbar vertebra.

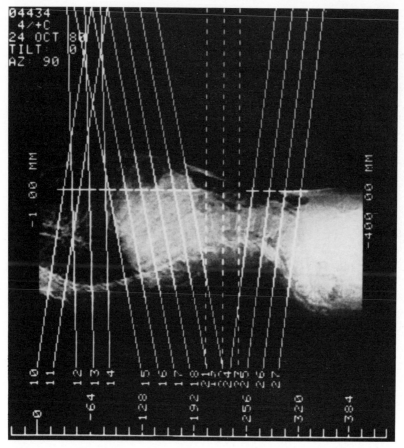

Fig. 2.4. Lateral Scout view and cursor lines. Boy, 13 years, with pronounced kyphosis and lordosis. Cursor lines annotate the levels of the sections, as well as the angle of the gantry, perpendicular to most sections of the spine. The angling of the gantry is insufficient to accommodate the lordosis in the lumbosacral region (sections 26–27).

The Image

Window Setting

The Metrizamide as well as the surrounding bone have high attenuation values, causing an over-range with "blooming" of the image on the screen. To diminish this, it is essential to use a wide window width and a high window level. It is often also valuable to reverse the color scale to black on white, as structures with low attenuation, for instance the cord and nerve roots, then appear white, and thus the unavoidable over-range on the screen makes these structures appear enlarged and more clearly visible (Fig. 2.6a). The Metrizamide–CSF solution and the bone that appears bloomed using the conventional color scale (white on black), obliterates the details of the cord and roots (Fig. 2.6b). If the General Electric CT/T 8800 ReView program for high spatial resolution and contrast discrimination (see below) is used, the conventional color scale (white on black) is satisfactory.

It should be noted that the apparent size of the cord and the thecal sac obtained with the window settings described here may not represent the true size. To get accurate measurements a special window setting is necessary, as shown by Seibert et al. (1981) (see Chap. 3).

High Spatial Resolution and Contrast Discrimination (ReView)

To enhance the spatial resolution and contrast discrimination the General Electric CT/T 8800 provides a computer program giving target reconstruction of the raw data obtained during the scanning. This target reconstruction is, according to Blumenfeld (1980), a "back projection of a part of the total field of view on very small pixels together with appropriate modifications in the convolution kernel and other parts of the reconstruction algorithm".

The target reconstruction combined with double-pass reconstruction for correction of the bone-hardening effect on the spine is called "ReView" in the General Electric Medical Systems, and it increases the spatial resolution and contrast discrimination considerably (Fig. 2.7). In this ReView program the window scale is extended to range between −1000 and +3000 Hounsfield units. As mentioned above, the raw data obtained at the initial standard scanning is used and thus the ReView means no additional radiation dose. The disadvantage is the complexity of the computer program—with the programs available today the review time for each image is 60–90 s. However, with improving technique, in the near future this time will be considerably diminished, and probably this and other high resolution image systems will replace the standard lower resolution image of today in most CT machines.

Image Reconstruction to Planes Angled to the Initial Transaxial Section

With the aid of the computer, a block of data may be chosen from each image of a series of continuous transaxial sections. From this block an image at any angle to the initial transaxial sections may be obtained. Such a reconstructed image may be regarded as a slice cut from a stack of axial sections and viewed from the side (Ullrich and Kieffer, 1980). The most often used reconstruction planes are the sagittal and coronal (Fig. 2.8), which often are helpful in providing a better three-dimensional impression of a lesion. Oblique reconstruction planes are less commonly used. However, the plane of the reconstructed image may be chosen to parallel the vertebral end plate, which is valuable for instance when the tilting of the gantry is not sufficient to overcome the natural lordosis or a pronounced kyphosis, as well as in cases of scoliosis (Hirschy et al., 1981).

To obtain detailed information from the reconstruction, the transaxial sections should be 5 mm thick or less, which means a relatively higher radiation dose to the patient.

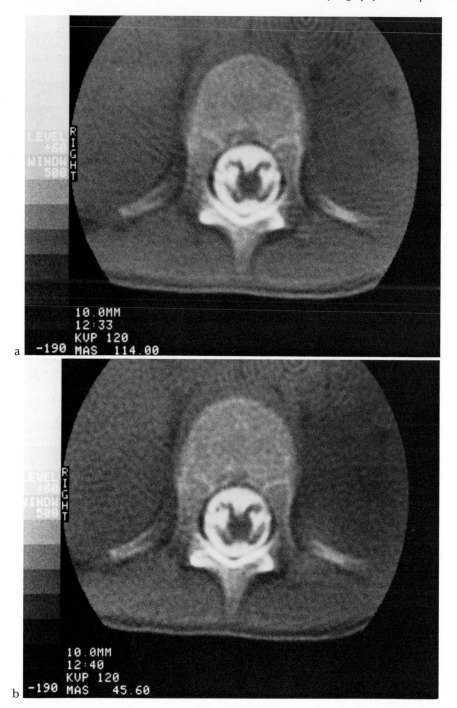

Fig. 2.5. Low-dose CT. Girl, 6 years, T12. The images are obtained with General Electric CT/T ReView program for high resolution. The same anatomic section through the conus has been scanned with three different radiation doses. All three scans were performed using 120 kV and 10-mm thickness of the section. (a) 114 mAs (700 mR), (b) 46 mAs (300 mR), and (c) 23 mAs (150 mR). The lowest dose provides detailed information on the spinal canal, although the electronic noise is more pronounced. Note the conus and the roots.

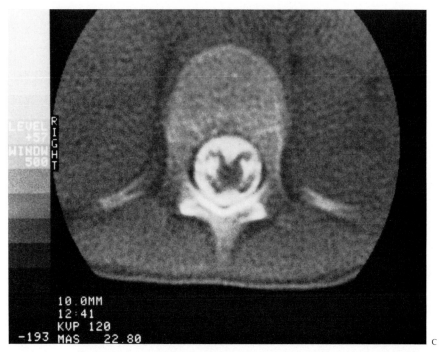

LEVEL
+57
WINDOW
500

R
I
G
H
T

10.0MM
12:41
KVP 120
-193 MAS 22.80

c

Fig. 2.5. (*Continued*)

Direct Coronal Sections

Although the programs for reconstructions are steadily improving, the images still do not give complete and accurate detailed information. As mentioned above, the relatively higher radiation dose needed must also be considered.

Direct coronal sections provide a much better spatial resolution than the reconstruction. This method has recently been described for body scanning (Kaiser and Veiga-Pires, 1981) and we have found it valuable in the examination of the pediatric spinal canal (Kaiser et al., 1981). To obtain direct coronal sections, the child is sat in the gantry hole with a slightly flexed spine, or is placed in the lateral decubitus position across the examination table, the long axis of the body being parallel to the plane of the gantry (Fig. 2.9). The patient's head, being outside the CT table, may be supported by a small plate, or better, by the radiologist's hands. Using the largest scanning circle, 9.6-s scanning time, and 10-mm thickness of the sections, coronal images of the spine and spinal canal of very high accuracy will be obtained (Fig. 2.10). However, this method can be used only for children up to the age of 5 years in most CT scanners, because of the small gantry holes.

As described by Harwood-Nash and Fitz (1980), direct coronal sections may be obtained of the occipitocervical region and the upper cervical vertebrae if the patient is positioned supine, with a pillow beneath the shoulders and the neck maximally extended (see Fig. 3.2).

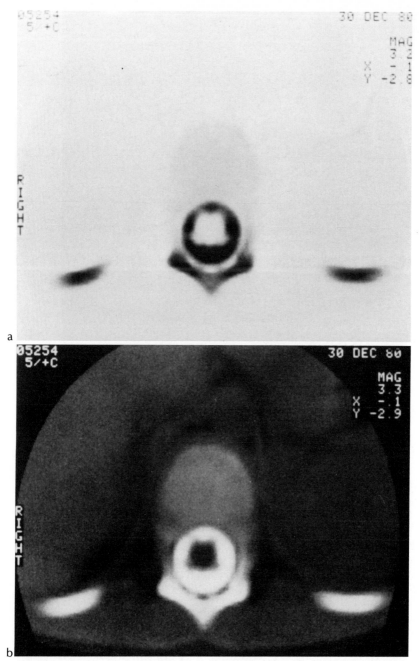

Fig. 2.6. Window width and color reversal. Examples of window setting, with standard resolution images. Boy, 4 years, L1. Transaxial section of the conus, with emerging roots.
(a) The wide window width and high window level diminish the over-range in the image. The reversed color scale (black on white) makes the cord and roots appear white and the surrounding CSF–Metrizamide solution, black. The unavoidable over-range will then apparently enlarge the cord and roots, making them more clearly visible.
(b) Same image as in (a), with standard color scale (white on black). Now the CSF–Metrizamide solution appears white and the over-range partly obliterates the cord and roots, these structures appearing considerably smaller and less visible than in (a).

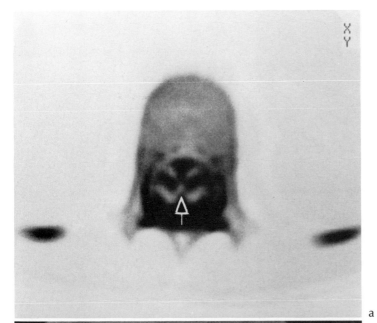

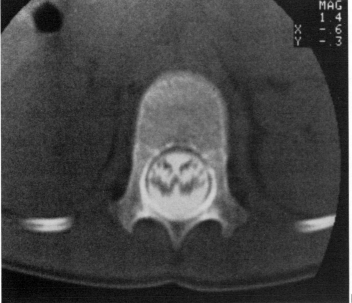

Fig. 2.7. Standard and high resolution images. Boy, 4 years, L1. Comparison between (a) standard resolution and (b) high resolution image obtained after ReView. Transaxial section through the tip of the conus and the beginning of the filum terminale.
(a) The standard resolution image shows the tip of the conus (*arrow*) and what appear to be two pairs of roots emerging from this tip. The color scale has been reversed to give optimal visual conditions.
(b) The high resolution image reveals the individual nerve roots of the cauda equina, and the better spatial resolution and contrast discrimination also allows evaluation of the extradural space as well as the skeleton and the soft tissues.

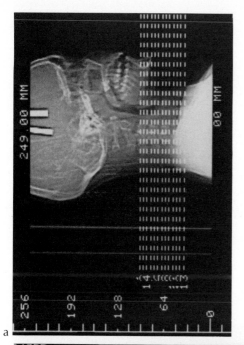

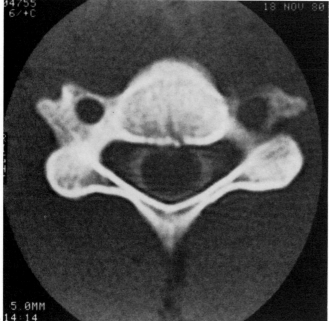

Fig. 2.8. Reconstruction in the coronal and sagittal planes. Girl, 14 years, with neck injury.
(a) The Scout view with cursor lines annotates continuous transaxial sections at the level C3–C7.
(b) A fracture of the C4 vertebral body is present. Metrizamide has been injected into the subarachnoid space.
(c) Proposed reformat sections through the neck in coronal and sagittal planes set by the cursor lines.
(d) The coronal and sagittal sections as indicated in (c). Note the posterior dislocation of the posterior wall of the C3 body with impingement on the thecal sac (*arrow*).

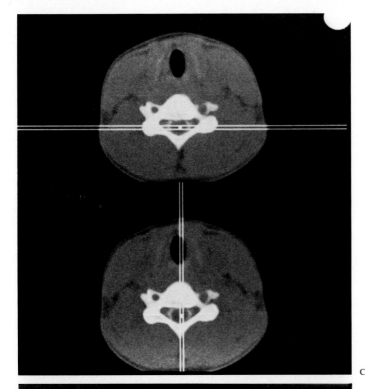

c

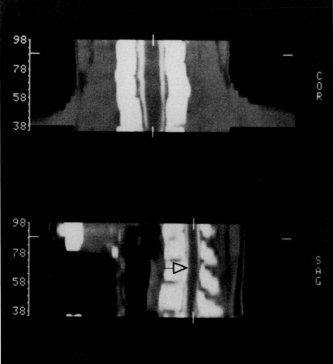

d

Fig. 2.8. (*Continued*)

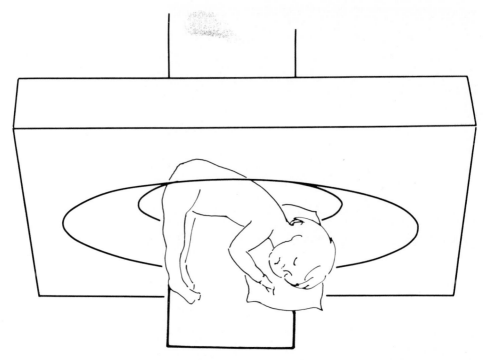

Fig. 2.9. Direct coronal CT. Drawing of the position of the patient for direct coronal sections. The patient is positioned decubitus on the table, with the long axis of the body parallel to the gantry.

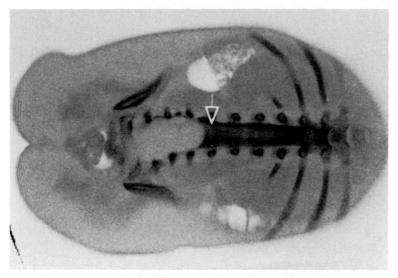

Fig. 2.10. Direct coronal CT. Girl, 9 months. Direct coronal sections through the spinal canal. Metrizamide has been injected in the thecal sac and the highly detailed image shows the low cord entering the large lumbosacral intraspinal lipoma (*arrow*) (reversed color scale).

References

Amundsen P (1977) Metrizamide in cervical myelography. Acta Radiol [Suppl] (Stockh) 355: 85–97

Anderson RE, Osborn AG (1977) Efficacy of simple sedation for pediatric computed tomography. Radiology 124: 739–740

Blumenfeld SM (1980) Physical principles of high resolution CT with the General Electric CT/T 8800. In: Post MJD (ed), Radiographic evaluation of the spine. Masson, New York, pp 295–307

Fitz CR, Harwood-Nash DC, Barry JF, Byrd SE (1977) Pediatric myelography with Metrizamide. Acta Radiol [Suppl] (Stockh) 355: 182–192

Harwood-Nash, Fitz CR (1980) Computed tomography and the pediatric spine: computed tomographic Metrizamide myelography in children. In: Post MJD (ed), Radiographic evaluation of the spine. Masson, New York, pp 4–33

Hirschy JC, Leue WM, Berninger WH, Hamilton RH, Abbott GF (1981) CT of the lumbosacral spine: importance of tomographic planes parallel to vertebral end plate. AJR 136: 47–52

Kaiser MC, Pettersson H, Harwood-Nash DC, Fitz CR, Armstrong E (1981) A direct coronal CT-mode of the spine in infants and children. AJNR 2: 465–466

Kaiser MC, Veiga-Pires JA (1981) Sitting position variation of direct longitudino-axial (semi-coronal) mode in CT scanning. ROEFO 134: 97–99

Pettersson H, Fitz CR, Harwood-Nash DC, Chuang S, Armstrong E (1982) Adverse effects to myelography with Metrizamide in infants, children and adolescents. I. General and CNS effects. Acta Radiol [Diagn] (Stockh) in press

Pettersson H, Fitz CR, Harwood-Nash DC, Chuang S, Armstrong E (1982) Adverse effects to myelography with Metrizamide in infants, children and adolescents. II. Local damage caused by the needle puncture and Metrizamide injection. Acta Radiol [Diagn] (Stockh) in press

Resjö IM, Harwood-Nash DC, Fitz CR, Chuang S (1979) Normal cord in infants and children examined with computed tomographic Metrizamide myelography. Radiology 130: 691–696

Rohrer RH, Sprawls P Jr, Mitler WB Jr, Weens HS (1964) Radiation doses received in myelographic examinations. Radiology 82: 106–112

Seibert CE, Barnes JE, Dreisbach JN, Swanson WB, Heck RJ (1981) Accurate CT measurement of the spinal cord using Metrizamide: physical factors. AJNR 2: 75–78

Sortland O, Hovind K (1977) Myelography with Metrizamide in children. Acta Radiol [Suppl] (Stockh) 355: 211–220

Tourtellotte WW, Henderson WG, Tucher RP, Gilland O, Walker JE, Kokman E (1972) A randomized, double blind clinical trial comparing the 22 versus the 26 gauge needle in the production of the post-lumbar puncture syndrome in normal individuals. Headache 12: 73–78

Ullrich CG, Kieffer SA (1980) Computed tomographic evaluation of the lumbar spine: quantitative aspects and sagittal-coronal reconstruction. In: Post MJD (ed) Radiographic evaluation of the spine. Masson, New York, pp 88–107

Chapter 3

The Normal Spine and Spinal Cord

The old adage of "know the normal, recognize the abnormal, and understand the pathology" holds true for CT of the spine as it does in all other fields of diagnostic imaging. The standard radiographic anatomy of the spine and spinal cord is well known, but high resolution CT and CTMM have added a new dimension to the imaging of these structures, and hence a thorough description of the normal anatomy is necessary before discussing pathologic changes.

The anatomy of the spine and its contents in children is subject to a dynamic change during growth until the adult stage is reached. There is not only a change in the shape and size of the vertebral bodies, the bony spinal canal, the dural sac, and the cord; with increasing age there is also a progressive change in the relationships between the relative size of these different structures.

The Spinal Column and Canal

In the examination of the spine at different ages, three important considerations emerge:

1. The altering shape of the spinal column itself, following the development of the normal cervical and lumbar lordosis, as well as the thoracic kyphosis.

2. The anatomy of the developing vertebral body, with growth of the different ossification centers, and subsequent fusion of the cartilagenous junctions between these centers.

3. The alteration with age of the shape and size of the spinal canal at different levels relative to the vertebral body at the corresponding level.

Shape of the Spinal Column

The infant's spine is relatively straight from occiput to coccyx. When the child begins to sit and walk, the cervical and lumbar lordosis as well as the thoracic kyphosis appear. This is important to bear in mind when choosing the gantry angles for the CTMM examination. Thus, in the small child the CT sections perpendicular to the table will be perpendicular to the spine, while in the older child the normal lordosis and kyphosis must be considered and CT sections perpendicular to each vertebra obtained, as has been described in Chap. 2.

Vertebral Ossification

During fetal life the vertebral bodies initially are formed from eight cartilagenous centers, which at birth usually have fused to one or possibly two ossification centers. If there are two centers, they are normally divided by a sagittal or coronal cleft. The neural arch is ossified from one center on each side (Fig. 3.1).

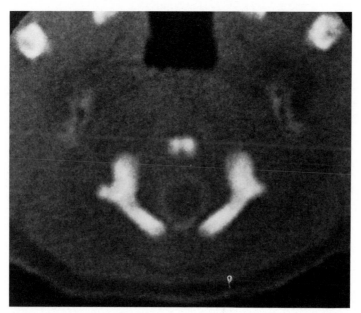

Fig. 3.1. Normal cervical spine. Section through the odontoid process of C2 and the posterior arches of C1 in a newborn girl. The anterior arch of C1 is not yet ossified. Note the normal sagittal cleft between the two ossification centers of the odontoid, and the normal wide cartilagenous junction in the midline posteriorly. There is a small amount of Metrizamide in the subarachnoid space. The cervical cord is round and centrally placed.

The number of ossification centers in the C1 vertebra varies in the anterior and posterior arches. Thus the anterior arch may ossify from one to four centers, and there might be an additional small center posteriorly in the midline between the two ossification centers of the posterior arches.

The odontoid process may be quite small in infancy, and normally contains two ossification centers, divided by a sagittal "cleft" and positioned symmetrically within the C1 arch (Fig. 3.1). The tip of the odontoid ossifies from one or two separate centers. The relationship between the occipital condyles and the C1, as well as between the C1 and C2 vertebrae, is often best seen in the coronal view (Fig. 3.2).

The lower cervical vertebrae in infancy ossify from a small composite center in the vertebral body, and from two C-shaped ossification centers in the pedicle–lamina complexes; with very small transverse processes. During the first years of life the pedicles become thicker and the transverse processes and the foramina transversaria are completely formed at approximately 3 years of age (Fig. 3.3). The

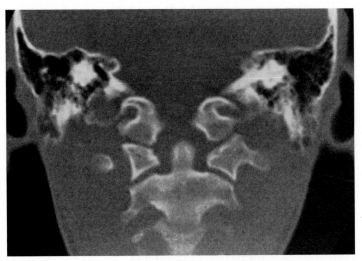

Fig. 3.2. Normal cervical spine, direct coronal section. Boy, 17 years. The relationships between C2, the odontoid process, the lateral masses of C1 and the occiput are clearly outlined.

lamina becomes longer and thinner in later childhood. In the thoracic region the pedicles are longer than the lamina (Fig. 3.4), in contrast to the lumbar spine, where the pedicles are thick and of the same length as the lamina (Fig. 3.5).

The ossified parts of the pedicles and lamina in the sacrum are quite small in

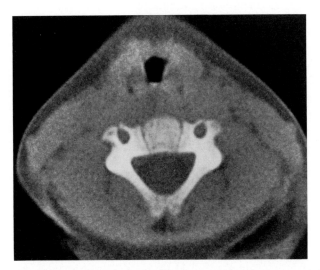

Fig. 3.3. Normal cervical spine. In a 2-year-old boy the neurocentral synchondrosis of C4 as well as the junction between the posterior arches is very narrow. The foramina transversaria are almost completely surrounded by bone.

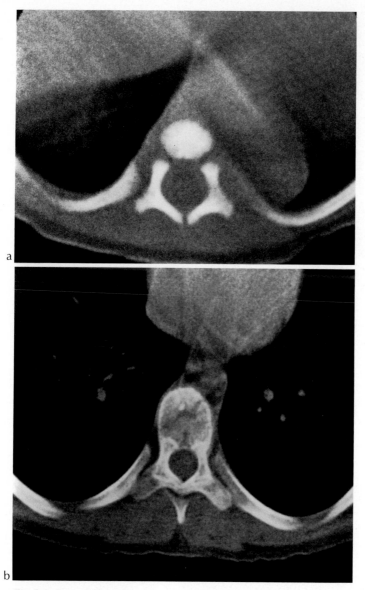

Fig. 3.4. Normal thoracic spine.
(a) T9 in a newborn girl. The neurocentral synchondrosis is wide. The spinal canal is slightly larger in the transverse diameter than the ossified part of the vertebral body.
(b) T8 in an 11 year old boy. The neurocentral synchondrosis is closed, and there is a dense area at the site of the junction. The spinal canal is small compared with the vertebral body. The pedicles are thin.

infancy and during the first years of life, the heavy buttressing of these structures appearing at about the age of 5. The intervertebral foramina, the alae and the sacroiliac joints are *symmetric*, and the sacroiliac joints are wide in the infant and small child (Fig. 3.6).

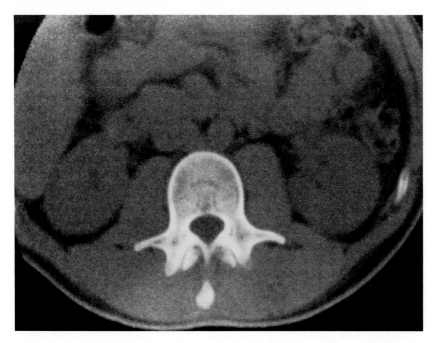

Fig. 3.5. Normal lumbar spine. L2 in a 7-year-old boy. The neurocentral synchondrosis is closed. The spinal canal is small compared with the vertebral body and is triangular. The pedicles are short and thick.

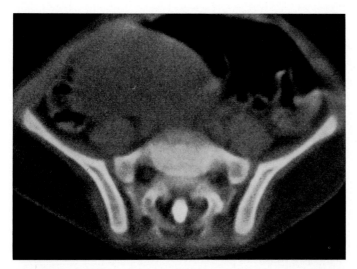

Fig. 3.6. Normal sacral spine. S1 in a 4-year-old boy. The ossification of the alae has begun, but the cartilagenous part of the sacroiliac joint is still wide. There is total symmetry in the side-to-side aspect.

The Cartilagenous Junctions

The cartilagenous junctions between the ossification centers are prominent in the infant and small child, and disappear during growth. The following cartilagenous junctions are normally seen:

1. As stated above, there might be a sagittal "cleft" in the ossification center of the vertebral body at birth. This cleft normally fuses before 6 months of age. The junctions between the ossification centers of the anterior arch of the C1 vertebra normally disappear before the age of 3 years. The odontoid process may be ossified from one or two ossification centers (Fig. 3.1), these being fused to each other and to the C2 vertebra during the first year of life.

2. The neurocentral junction between the vertebral body and the neural arch is wide in the infant and small child (Figs. 3.4a, 3.11) and progressively ossifies to disappear at about 4 years of age. Often a remnant of increased bony density at the fusion site may persist to late childhood or adolescence (Figs. 3.4b, 3.12).

3. The junction of the two halves of the spinous processes may be seen in all the vertebrae at birth. They progressively ossify with increasing age, the latest to ossify being those at C1 and L5, which close at approximately the age of 5 years. As stated above, there might be an additional ossification center appearing in the junction between the two posterior arches of the C1 vertebra. The cartilagenous junction between the posterior arches should never be regarded as spina bifida (Figs. 3.1, 3.4a).

The Spinal Canal

Not only the size and shape of the spinal canal change with increasing age, but also the size of the canal relative to the size of the vertebral bodies. The normal anatomy and size of the vertebral bodies and spinal canal as appearing at CT has been thoroughly investigated in adults (Coin et al., 1978; Hammerschlag et al., 1976; Lee et al., 1978; Sheldon et al., 1977; Ullrich and Kieffer, 1980), while few reports concerning children are on record (Harwood-Nash and Fitz, 1980). The absolute size of the spinal canal increases until about the age of 16, when the adult size is obtained. There is a wide variation in size among children of the same age, as there is in adults.

In infants and small children, the transverse diameter of the canal is wider than that of the vertebral body at all levels of the spine (Figs. 3.1, 3.4a, 3.7). From the age of 6–8 years, the transverse diameter of the cervical canal is only slightly larger than, or of the same size as, that of the cervical vertebral body, as it is in adults (Figs. 3.7, 3.9). At this same age the thoracic canal is smaller than the vertebral body, as it is in the lumbar area, where the canal is smallest in relation to the vertebral body (Figs. 3.4b, 3.7).

The shape of the spinal canal is subject to considerable change during growth. In infancy and early childhood the cervical canal is oval with the large diameter transversely, the thoracic canal oval with the large diameter in the sagittal plane, and the lumbar canal oval as in the cervical. The sacral canal is wider in the transverse diameter, and oriented in a shallow rounded triangle with the apex posteriorly. With increasing age the shape of the whole canal becomes more triangulated, with the apex posteriorly. A survey of the changing size and shape of the vertebral bodies and spinal canal at different levels of the spine and at different ages, is given in Fig. 3.7.

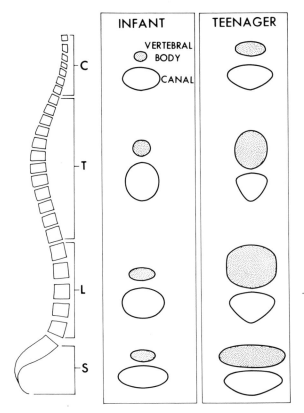

Fig. 3.7. Normal infant/child size relationship. Schematic drawing of the size-relationship between the ossified part of the vertebral bodies and spinal canal in different ages and at different levels of the spine.

The Dural Sac and Spinal Cord

With high resolution CTMM, it is possible to visualize detailed anatomy of the cord itself, the nerve roots emerging from the cord at all levels, each root within the cauda equina, and the filum terminale, as well as the anterior and posterior spinal arteries. The combination of conventional MM and high resolution CTMM is today the only method available that provides this detailed information of the size, shape, and position of the intrathecal structures in vivo. Conventional radiologic examination with previously used contrast media provided much less anatomic detail, and exploration at surgery or autopsy means an opened dura with deranged fluid dynamics in the dural sac and ensuing change in position of the intrathecal structures.

As with the spinal canal, the size and shape of the dural sac and the size and position of the spinal cord change between different levels of the spine and between different ages. Regardless of these changes, *absolute symmetry* from one side to the other is the rule.

Shape

At the foramen magnum, where the medulla oblongata merges into the cervical cord, the vertebral arteries may be seen on both sides, as may the hypoglossal nerve (Fig. 3.8). At this and at the C1 level the cord is rounded and centrally placed in the canal and in the subarachnoid space (Fig. 3.8). Lower down in the cervical canal,

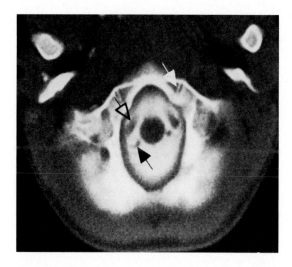

Fig. 3.8. Normal cervical cord, Girl, 5 years. At the foramen magnum the cord is round and centrally placed. The vertebral arteries (*open arrow*) are seen on both sides as are the hypoglossal nerves (*black arrow*). Note the ex-occipital synchondrosis between the basis occiput and ex-occiput (*white arrow*).

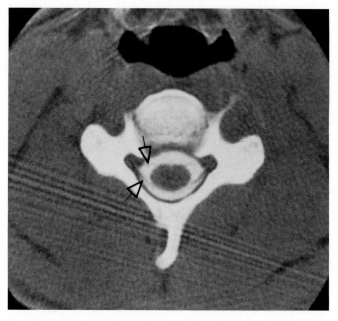

Fig. 3.9. Normal cervical cord. In a 14-year-old boy, the spinal canal at C4 has a larger transverse diameter than the vertebral body. The cord as well as the dural sac is oval with a large transverse diameter. The emerging nerve roots (*arrows*) as well as the root sleeves are well visible.

the dural sac as well as the cord becomes oval, with the larger diameter in the transverse direction. The anterior and posterior cervical roots are clearly seen, as are the emerging root sleeves (Fig. 3.9). In the infant, however, until about the age of 6 months, the subarachnoid space and cord are more rounded throughout the cervical region (Fig. 3.1).

At the cervico-thoracic junction the cord is still centrally placed in the sub-arachnoid space, but becomes relatively smaller. At the level of T3 and below, the dural sac is slightly oval, the large diameter in the sagittal plane, and the cord, still smaller, situated close to the *anterior* wall of the sac (Fig. 3.10). This is due to

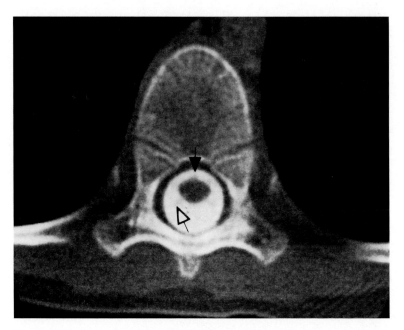

Fig. 3.10. Normal thoracic cord. T4 in an 8-year-old boy. The dural sac is slightly oval with the large diameter in the AP direction. The cord is small, and anteriorly placed in the subarachnoid space and spinal canal. The nerve roots (*open arrow*) and the anterior spinal artery (*black arrow*) are visualized. Note the open neurocentral synchondrosis.

kyphosis of the thoracic spine and is the only area in which the cord is normally anteriorly placed in the canal. However, before the normal lordosis and kyphosis have developed in the infant, the cord is central in this region. In the thoracic area, the extradural space, containing more fat, is larger than in the cervical area.

At the T10–T11 level, the cord insidiously widens to form the bulbous conus and becomes more centrally placed within the canal and subarachnoid space. The anterior and posterior roots emerging from this area are large, as are the anterior and posterior spinal arteries (Fig. 3.11). At this level and downwards, the cord and roots have the same configuration regardless of age. At the L1–L2 level, the conus narrows to form the filum terminale (Fig. 3.12), and at this level all the nerve roots forming the cauda equina are clearly visible (Fig. 3.13). The normal level of the tip of the conus changes with age, but has not been determined for all ages. Normally

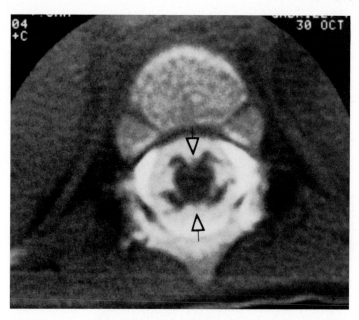

Fig. 3.11. Normal conus. L1 in a 1-year-old boy. The emerging nerve roots are normally thick. Note the anterior and posterior spinal arteries (*arrows*). Note also that there has been a considerable leak of contrast medium into the extradural space through the needle puncture site. This amount of leakage will make assessment of the cord and roots at conventional myelography difficult, but does not disturb the CTMM appearance. On the contrary, it outlines the thickness of the dura.

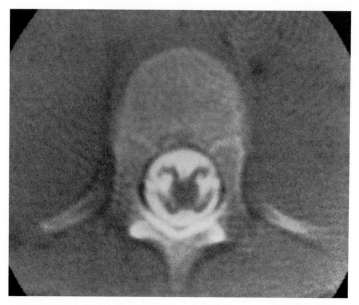

Fig. 3.12. The lower conus. Mid L1 in a 6-year-old girl. As the conus is giving off the nerve roots that will form the cauda equina, it is tapering to merge into the filum terminale.

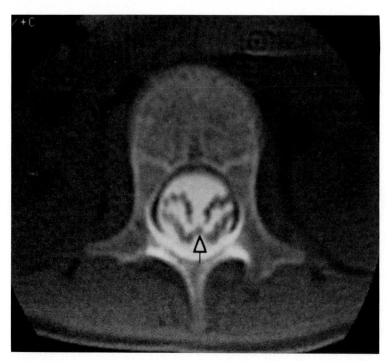

Fig. 3.13. Normal cord, the tip of the conus. Same patient as in Fig. 3.11, 20 mm further down (L1–L2 level). The tip of the conus is merging into the filum terminale (*arrow*). The nerve roots, each visualized, will form the cauda equina and are collected in symmetric pairs on both sides. Note the increased bony density at the site of the previous neurocentral synchondrosis.

the tip of the conus is at the L1–L2 interspace at the age of 2 months (Harwood-Nash and Fitz, 1976). However, in infants the tip of the conus may be situated at the L2–L3 disc space without any pathologic significance, and in our experience, by the age of 12 years the tip should be at or above the mid-L2 level.

Below the tip of the conus, the roots of the cauda equina as well as the filum terminale are situated in the posterior half of the dural sac in a V-shaped or crescentic collection (Fig. 3.14). At the low lumbar and the sacral region the filum terminale is usually too thin to be visualized (Fig. 3.15). Each root is visualized in the cauda equina, the sacral roots being situated medially and the lumbar, laterally.

The position of the cord and nerve roots within the subarachnoid space is not changed with changing position of the patient, as in flexion or extension of the spine. This is probably due to the cord being fixed by the nerves and the dentate ligaments.

Size

The apparent dimensions of structures in the CT image are relatively insensitive to window width settings, while the window level has an important effect (Koehler et al., 1979). This was also observed by Resjö et al. (1979) in the only report on the normal size of the cord in children, as seen at CTMM. They used a very high window level and wide window width to avoid measurement errors.

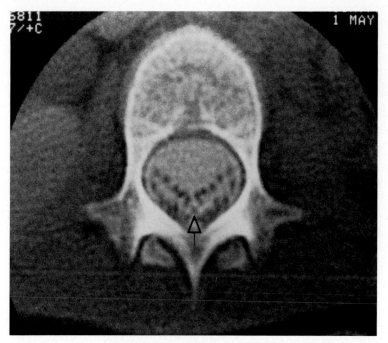

Fig. 3.14. Normal cauda equina. L3 in a 4-year-old boy. The nerve roots are arranged in a symmetric V or crescentic shape and the filum terminale is clearly visible in the midline (*arrow*). The sacral roots are aligned medial to the lumbar roots.

Recently, Seibert et al. (1981) have shown experimentally that the window level greatly influences the measurement values of the size of the cord, whereas the window width does not. The appropriate window level for size measurements is the mean between the attenuation values for the Metrizamide in the subarachnoid space and for the cord. The measurements are most accurately performed with a narrow window width (20–40 Hounsfield units).

Table 3.1 gives the size of the cord at different levels in different ages. These values were obtained from 45 patients in whom both MM and CTMM were performed, and each examination was considered normal. Twenty-three patients were examined on an Ohio-Nuclear Delta 50 scanner, with a measurement error of about 1.0 mm., and 22 patients on a General Electric CT/T 8800 scanner, with a measurement error of about 0.5 mm. As the size of the cord was measured at all the recorded levels in each of only a few patients, the number of measurements at each level and in each age group does not allow any extensive statistical analysis. However, from the Table 3.1 it is clear that the cord increases in size most rapidly during the first months of life, while after about the age of 6 months the rate of increase of the size is much slower. This is probably due to the rapid myelinization occurring during the first months after birth. The measurement values reported here are in accordance with the studies performed by Nordqvist (1964), who did a roentgenographic postmortem study of the sagittal diameters of the spinal cord in different age groups. The values are also in accordance with those obtained by Resjö et al. (1979).

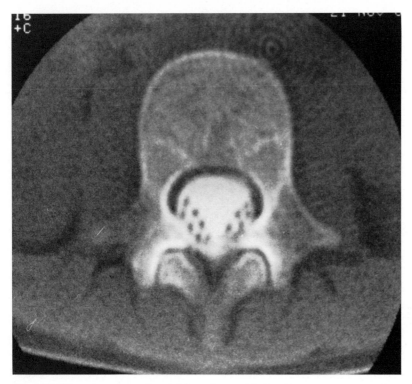

Fig. 3.15. Normal cauda equina. L5 in a 6-year-old girl. The nerve roots are fewer and the filum terminale is not visible.

From Table 3.1 it is also clear that the range is fairly large in several levels and age groups, and thus, in most cases, the morphology of the cord, its symmetry, and its size compared to the subarachnoid space and the spinal canal is more important than the absolute measurement values.

Attenuation Values

Without injection of any contrast medium, the dural sac and its contents appear of a homogeneous density within the spinal canal, enclosed by the epidural fat. However, the cervical cord at the C1–C2 level may be seen within the subarachnoid space (Ethier et al., 1979).

In children, the attenuation values of the cord before injection of contrast medium varies between 30 and 35 Hounsfield units (Harwood-Nash and Fitz, 1980). After intravenous contrast medium injection (Hypaque 60%, 3 ml/kg body wt.) the attenuation value of the cord may increase by about 10 Hounsfield units. Also the attenuation value of the epidural space increases after contrast medium injection, probably because of contrast-containing blood in the extradural venous plexuses.

When Metrizamide is injected into the subarachnoid space, there may be an increase of the attenuation value of the cord of about 30 Hounsfield units

(Harwood-Nash and Fitz, 1980; Isherwood et al., 1977). This represents an alternative route of absorption of the Metrizamide, probably in the Virchow–Robin spaces; most of the contrast medium follows the CSF circulation and is absorbed intracranially.

Table 3.1. Normal cord diameters at different levels and ages as measured at CTMM. The numbers give the mean values and (within brackets) range, expressed in millimeters.

Age \ Level	C3 AP	C3 Lat	C–T AP	C–T Lat	T6 AP	T6 Lat
0 < 6 months (n = 4)	5.0 (4.5–5.5)	6.5 (6.0–7.0)	5.0 (4.5–5.5)	6.0 (5.5–6.5)	3.5 (3.0–3.5)	3.5 (3.0–3.5)
6 months < 2 years (n = 7)	7.0 (6.5–8.0)	9.5 (8.5–10.5)	6.0 (5.5–6.5)	8.5 (7.5–9.0)	5.0 (4.5–5.5)	6.0 (5.0–7.0)
2 < 6 years (n = 7)	7.0 (6.0–7.5)	10.0 (9.5–11.0)	6.0 (5.0–7.0)	8.5 (6.5–11.0)	5.0 (4.5–6.0)	6.0 (5.5–8.0)
6 < 12 years (n = 9)	7.5 (7.0–8.0)	10.5 (9.5–11.5)	6.0 (5.5–6.0)	8.5 (7.5–9.5)	5.5 (5.0–6.0)	7.0 (6.5–8.0)
12 < 18 years (n = 15)	7.5 (6.5–8.0)	11.5 (11.0–13.5)	6.5 (6.0–6.5)	9.0 (8.0–9.5)	6.0 (5.5–6.0)	7.5 (7.5–8.0)

Table 3.1. (continued)

Age \ Level	Conus AP	Conus Lat
0 < 6 months (n = 4)	4.0 (4.0–4.5)	5.0 (4.5–5.5)
6 months < 2 years (n = 7)	6.5 (5.5–7.0)	7.5 (6.5–9.0)
2 < 6 years (n = 7)	7.0 (6.5–7.5)	8.5 (8.0–9.0)
6 < 12 years (n = 9)	8.0 (7.0–8.5)	9.5 (9.0–9.5)
12 < 18 years (n = 15)	8.0 (7.0–9.0)	9.5 (8.0–11.0)

References

Coin C, Keranen VJ, Pennink M, Ahmad WD (1978) Computerized tomography of the spine and its contents. Neuroradiology 16: 271–272

Ethier R, King DG, Melancon D, Bélanger G, Taylor S, Thompson C (1979) Development of high resolution computed tomography of the spinal cord. J Comput Assist Tomogr 3: 433–438

Hammerschlag SB, Wolpert SM, Carter BL (1976) Computed tomography of the spinal canal. Radiology 121: 361–367

Harwood-Nash DC, Fitz CR (1976) Neuroradiology in infants and children. CV Mosby, St. Louis

Harwood-Nash DC, Fitz CR (1980) Computed tomography and the pediatric spine: computed tomographic Metrizamide myelography in children. In: Post MJD (ed) Radiographic evaluation of the spine. Masson, New York, pp 4–33

Isherwood I, Fawcitt RA, St. Clair Forbes W, Nettle JR, Pullan BR (1977) Computer tomography of the spinal canal using Metrizamide. Acta Radiol [Suppl] (Stockh) 355: 299–305

Koehler PR, Anderson RE, Baxter B (1979) The effect of computed tomography viewer controls on anatomical measurements. Radiology 130: 189–194

Lee BC, Kazam E, Newman AD (1978) Computed tomography of the spine and spinal cord. Radiology 128: 95–102

Nordqvist L (1964) The sagittal diameter of the spinal cord and subarachnoid space in different age groups. A roentgenographic post mortem study. Acta Radiol [Suppl] (Stockh) 227

Resjö IM, Harwood-Nash DC, Fitz CR, Chuang S (1979) Normal cord in infants and children examined with computed tomographic Metrizamide myelography. Radiology 130: 691–696

Seibert CE, Barnes JE, Dreisbech JN, Swanson WB, Heck RJ (1981) Accurate CT measurement of the spinal cord using Metrizamide: physical factors. AJNR 2: 75–78

Sheldon JJ, Sersland T, Leborgne J (1977) Computed tomography of the lower lumbar vertebral column. Radiology 124: 113–118

Ullrich CG, Kieffer SA (1980) Computed tomographic evaluation of the lumbar spine: quantitative aspects and sagittal-coronal reconstruction. In: Post MJD (ed) Radiographic evaluation of the spine. Masson, New York, pp 88–107

Chapter 4
Spinal Dysraphism

The term "spinal dysraphism" was introduced by Lichtenstein (1940) to denote the occurrence and sequelae of defective fusion of the neural tube. Such dysraphism comprises a wide variety of abnormalities, varying in complexity and involving not only the structures derived from the ectodermal neural tube, but also tissues derived from entoderm and mesoderm. We prefer this overall term to spina bifida.

The dysraphic abnormalities may be occult, in which case no cutaneous abnormalities are directly visible; or manifest, revealed by cutaneous abnormalities such as a hairy or abnormally pigmented patch, vascular nevus, dermal sinus, lipoma, or even an overt meningocele or myelomeningocele.

The abnormalities of the spinal column may involve one or more of the vertebral bodies, which may be hypoplastic, or appear as hemivertebrae or cleft vertebrae, or there may be different defects in the vertebral segmentation. The abnormalities of the posterior neural arch include spina bifida, with asymmetric spinous components, and in more pronounced cases asymmetric and widely spread neural arches. There may also be laminar fusions at several vertebral levels.

The disorders of the formation of the spinal cord, nerve roots and thecal sac (myelomeningodysplasias) may be minor, only manifested as a wide dural sac or a thick filum with tethering of the cord. More pronounced changes include meningocele, myelomeningocele (to a considerable extent accompanied by a Chiari malformation), diastematomyelia, and syringohydromyelia. Overgrowth of tissue that was sequestered during fetal growth will result in excessive diffuse fatty tissue or developmental discrete mass lesions, such as dermoid, epidermoid, lipoma, or teratoma. Persistence of the transient open passage in the embryo between the yolk sac and the notochordal canal, will result in a neurenteric cyst.

There is no direct correlation between the degree of vertebral abnormality and the underlying neural abnormality. Thus a mild vertebral abnormality may be associated with pronounced disorganization of the neural tissues while a severe vertebral abnormality may be associated with only slight meningeal dysplasia without any other significant distortion of the neural tissues.

The CTMM appearance of the different myelomeningeal dysplasias and the different types of vertebral dysraphism will not be described separately, but in combination. This is a valid clinical and radiologic approach.

Widened Dural Sac

The widening of the dural sac probably represents the mildest form in the spectrum of myelomeningeal dysplasias, occurring in 3%–4% of all myelograms in large pediatric units (Harwood-Nash and Fitz, 1976). CTMM will reveal a wide sac in a wide spinal canal, without any other abnormalities.

Tethered Cord Syndrome

The tethered cord or fixed conus syndrome is common in pediatric neuroradiologic practice (Fitz and Harwood-Nash, 1975). In our series of 110 CTMMs performed in patients with dysraphism, a tethered cord was revealed in 62 (56%), in all cases accompanied by some degree of vertebral dysraphism (Table 4.1, p. 56).

The tethered cord and its associated abnormalities are clearly and accurately detected at CTMM (Harwood-Nash and Fitz, 1980; James and Oliff, 1977; Resjö et al., 1978). As mentioned in Chap. 3, the tip of the conus should be at or above the L2–L3 disc space in infants and at or above the mid-L2 level by the age of 12 years. The mildest form of the tethered cord may be revealed at the CT examination as a low position of a normal conus and a filum terminale that is thicker than 2 mm (Fitz and Harwood-Nash, 1979; Hoffman et al., 1976) (Fig. 4.1). In more pronounced cases, the cord itself may extend to a low lumbar or sacral level, *the low cord syndrome*. If the cord is thin, it must be differentiated from the thick filum by the nerve roots emerging from the cord. This is not possible to visualize with oil myelography, and barely with conventional MM, while at CTMM the emerging nerve roots are clearly visible (Fig. 4.2). Often lipomatous tissue is attached to the thick filum and the low cord (Fig. 4.2). Often a split cord is also

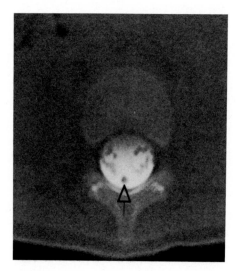

Fig. 4.1. Thick filum terminale. Girl, 1 year. The diameter of the filum terminale (*arrow*) at the level L4 is 3 mm, which is abnormal. The filum tethers the cord, and the position and symmetry of the nerve roots are slightly disturbed.

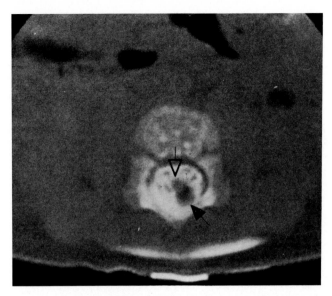

Fig. 4.2. Low cord. Boy, 2 months. At the level L4 the cord is thin (*open arrow*), but may be differentiated from a thick filum terminale by the emerging nerve roots. Lipomatous tissue is attached to the posterior left part of the cord (*black arrow*). Note the Metrizamide in the subcutaneous tissue, caused by leakage through the needle puncture canal.

tethered and if the splitting involves the caudal part of the cord, the two halves of the cord may extend to a low level of the spinal canal (Fig. 4.12), and there may be one or two thick filum terminale.

Meningocele

A *meningocele* is defined as an extension of the meninges outside the spinal canal. If the cord or other neural elements enter the meningocele or are attached to its wall, the lesion is defined as a *myelomeningocele*. A *lipomyelomeningocele* occurs where the lesion also contains lipomatous tissue. In *myelomeningocystocele* there is pronounced dilatation of the central canal, connected with the meningocele. *Intraspinal meningocele* is defined by us as a space-occupying lesion within the spinal canal, caused by herniation of the meninges through the wall of the dural sac but still contained within the spinal canal (Harwood-Nash and Fitz, 1976).

Conventional myelography of meningoceles might be technically difficult because of the large amounts of Metrizamide needed, and the problem of positioning. CTMM has the advantage that the Metrizamide can be inserted anywhere in the subarachnoid space, even via a cerebral ventricular shunt tube in a patient with hydrocephalus. If the aqueduct is patent the contrast medium will then enter the spinal subarachnoid space, and even a low iodine concentration will be seen at the CTMM in most cases.

In the dorsal meningoceles, or in the much less common ventral, or in the

intraspinal meningoceles the CTMM examination will reveal a CSF-filled meningeal cavity without any neural elements. The intraspinal meningocele may be seen
as a mass lesion within the spinal canal compressing the dural sac and cord
(Fig. 4.3). In the myelomeningocele the cord may be seen to enter the sac and

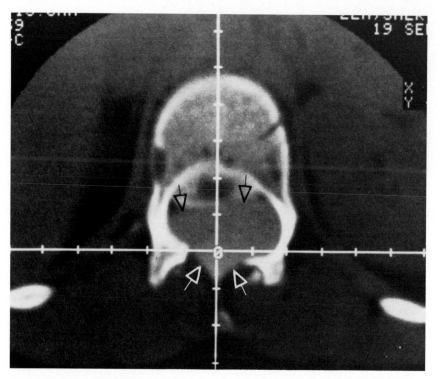

Fig. 4.3. Intraspinal meningocele. Girl, 16 years, T12. A large intraspinal meningocele (*arrows*) dorsal
to the dural sac compresses the dural sac as well as the cord. The concentration of Metrizamide is higher
in the dural sac than in the meningocele. (By courtesy of Dr. Killien, Seattle, Wash.)

neural elements may also appear as a neural placode at the wall of the lesion, from
which the nerve roots emerge, crossing the sac (Fig. 4.4).

In pronounced dysraphic cases, a large neural placode may be seen at the dorsal
wall of a wide sac, these changes being part of a spectrum of grotesque spinal
dysraphic abnormalities (Fig. 4.5).

The myelomeningoceles as well as other manifestations of spinal dysraphism are
often associated with abnormally positioned fatty tissue. This lipomatous tissue
may appear in the subcutaneous tissue, in the spinal muscles and in the extradural
portion of the spinal canal (Fig. 4.6), and it may extend into and around the cord,
the filum terminale, and the nerve roots (Fig. 4.2). This lipomatous tissue should
be differentiated from lipoma, which is a localized fibrolipomatous mass lesion
which, occurring in the spinal canal, may be associated with specific neurologic
symptoms identical with those of other developmental mass lesions (see Fig. 4.17).

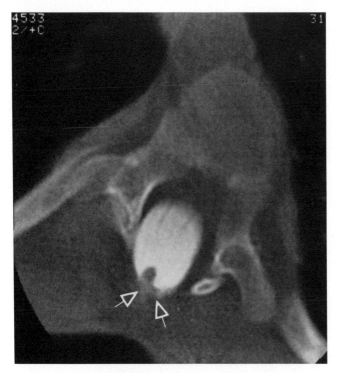

Fig. 4.4. Myelomeningocele. Boy, 12 years, L4. The posterior arches are widely spread apart, and an enlarged dural sac is herniated posteriorly. There is a small cord attached to the posterior wall of the sac, and the cord is adherent to a neural plaque (*arrows*). The nerve roots are emerging anteriorly from the cord through the enlarged sac.

Syringohydromyelia

Congenital dilatation of the central canal (hydromyelia) and cyst formation within the cord separate from the central canal (syringomyelia) may be difficult or impossible to distinguish both radiologically, clinically, and pathologically. Thus the combined term syringohydromyelia may better be used as first proposed by Gardner (1965). From this complex, cystic cavities of the cord caused by hemorrhage or associated with neoplasm should be excluded.

The cystic dilatation may involve only a part of the cord, often in the cervical or upper thoracic region, or it may involve the entire cord, which in these cases is often low. (The syringohydromyelia is one of three lesions that may extend through the cord in its entire length in childhood, the others being astrocytoma and teratoma.) In the dilated canal there may be irregular constrictions, giving the cavity an irregularly segmented or serrated appearance, as has been shown after direct puncture of contrast medium injection into the sac (Harwood-Nash and Fitz, 1976; Pettersson et al., 1982).

The CTMM examination often reveals a large spinal canal, as do the plain films. The large cystic dilatation of the cervical cord, often extending down through the thoracic region, was seen in 11 of our 23 cases of syringohydromyelia in which

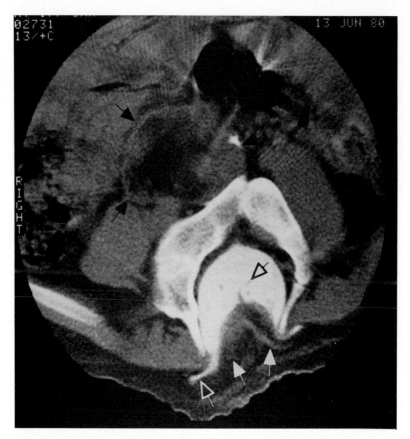

Fig. 4.5. Pronounced dysraphic abnormalities. Boy, 6 years, L5. There is a pronounced derangement of the vertebra, the vertebral body being very irregular and partly fused anteriorly, and the posterior arches being small and widely spread apart. The Metrizamide-filled arachnoid space fills the spinal canal, and extends to the fatty tissue on both sides dorsal to the vertebra (*white open arrow*). A large neural placode (*white arrow*) is bulging into the posterior part of the arachnoid space, and nerve roots (*black open arrow*) are seen in the subarachnoid space to be totally disorganized. In the abdomen there is probably a large teratoma (not surgically proven) (*black arrows*).

CTMM was performed (Fig. 4.7). The characteristic change in shape of the lesion during air myelography, with partial collapse of the cord in the upright position, as first described by Wickbom and Hanafee (1963) is not as commonly seen in MM. Probably the slight or absent changes in shape of the cord in MM reflect the naturally occurring gravity-induced deformation of the thin wall surrounding the cyst, while the pronounced changes seen in air myelography reflect the gravity-induced deformation following a considerable change of the normal fluid dynamics of the spinal canal, caused by the instillation of air.

As has been shown previously (Forbes and Isherwood, 1978; Resjö et al., 1979), the contrast medium may enter the syringohydromyeliac sac via the fourth ventricle and a patent obex. To assess this the patient should have a repeat CT scan about 4–5 h after the contrast medium injection. The attenuation value of the fluid in the sac may be more than 100 Hounsfield units at this repeat examination (Figs. 4.7, 4.9). It should be noted that a small increase in the attenuation values of the fluid of

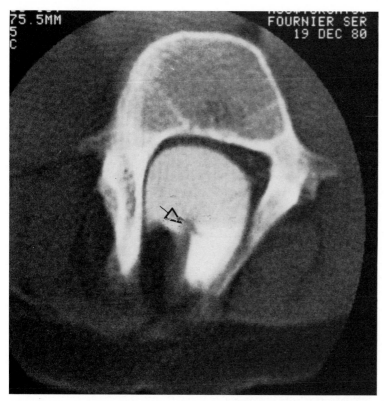

Fig. 4.6. Myelomeningocele, tethered cord, and lipomatous tissue. Boy, 10 years. At the L4 level a low, narrow cord (*arrow*) is adherent to lipomatous tissue, and the tissue bulges out dorsally into the spinal muscles.

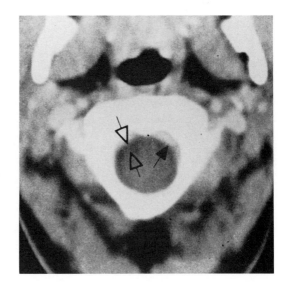

Fig. 4.7. Syringohydromyelia. Girl, 17 years, C1. In the cervical canal, the cord is markedly expanded, compressing the subarachnoid space to a thin Metrizamide-filled rim anteriorly and laterally (*black arrow*). Metrizamide has entered the large syringohydromyeliac sac although the concentration is much less than in the subarachnoid space. The dark area between the *two open arrows* outlines the thin wall of neural tissue, surrounding the cystic cavity.

the sac will also be seen even though the obex is closed. In these cases there is probably a diffusion of the contrast medium through the wall of the syringo-hydromyeliac sac. Ethier et al. (1979), using high resolution CT, described detection of the cystic cavity due to syringohydromyelia in the cervical cord without Metrizamide. However, in our opinion, if a syringohydromyelia appears as a cystic expansion that does not collapse and in which no Metrizamide enters through a patent obex, the differentiation from a cystic neoplasm may be difficult or impossible.

The syringohydromyelia may also appear as a flattened cord, most often in the cervical region. This appearance was seen in 12 of our 23 cases examined with CTMM. This cord has a decreased AP diameter and a slight increase in transverse diameter. The CTMM examination reveals that the anterior border of the cord is relatively straight, often with a small concave indentation in the midline (Figs. 4.8, 4.9). If examined in the decubitus position, the dependent part of the flattened cord might increase slightly in the AP diameter as described by Resjö et al. (1979). However the change in shape between the supine and decubitus position is very slight, as the cord is fixed by the dentate ligaments and the emerging nerve roots (McRae and Standen, 1966) (Figs. 4.8, 4.9).

A normal sized or atrophic or small cord containing a syringohydromyeliac sac, as described by Ethier et al. (1980) in adult subjects, was not seen in our cases.

Inadvertent puncture of the sac and ensuing Metrizamide injections will give a very dense opacification of the cystic cavity. CT sections through the fourth ventricle will then reveal if the obex is open. We have had one case in which the syringohydromyeliac sac was inadvertently punctured (Fig. 4.10). The patient had

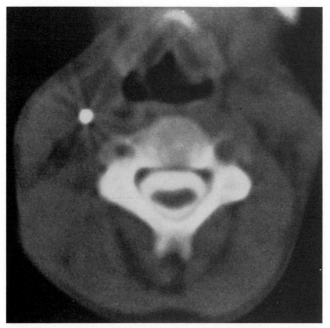

Fig. 4.8. Syringohydromyelia. Boy, 11 years, C4. The syringohydromyelia appears as a flattened cord with a slight indentation in the anterior midline, and there is a slight asymmetry between the left and right parts of the cord.

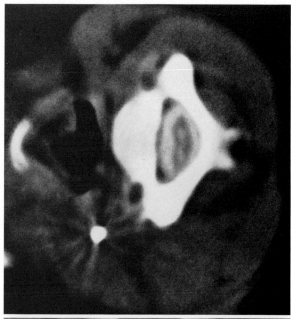

Fig. 4.9. Syringohydromyelia. Same patient and level as in Fig. 4.8. Repeat CT 5h later. Metrizamide with high concentration has entered the syringohydromyeliac cavity. The patient is positioned decubitus with the right side down, but this only to a very small degree changes the shape of the cord as compared with Fig. 4.8.

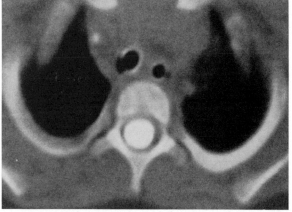

Fig. 4.10. Syringohydromyelia. Girl, 6 years, T4. Metrizamide has been injected directly into the sac at the L3–L4 level. The syringohydromyeliac cavity is opacified.

no unexpected discomfort at the examination, and there was no new neurologic disturbance during or after the procedure.

Syringohydromyelia is often accompanied by a Chiari malformation (see Fig. 4.18) and examination of the occipitocervical junction should always be performed in cases of syringohydromyelia using CTMM, wherein the low tonsils are readily demonstrated. Syringobulbia within a large brain stem is very rare.

Diastematomyelia

Diastematomyelia denotes a longitudinal split of the spinal cord extending over one or several vertebral levels, or rarely over multiple discrete levels, usually in the lower thoracic or upper lumbar area, although higher levels or the filum terminale might also be involved. The two parts of the cord may be situated in the dural sac, or may be separated by a bony, cartilagenous, or fibrous spur that protrudes into or through the sac. Diastematomyelia should be distinguished from the very rarely occurring diplomyelia which is a true duplication of the spinal cord, with two complete sets of nerve roots in two dural sacs, as well as from the still rarer total duplication of the spine itself.

The condition was previously considered to be rare, only a few cases being diagnosed ante mortem (Dale, 1969). More sophisticated neuroradiologic methods, including conventional MM, led to a higher frequency of the diagnosis, and in recent years there have been several reports on the accuracy of CT in examination of diastematomyelia (Lohkampf et al., 1978; Tadmor et al., 1977; Weinstein et al., 1975; Wolpert et al., 1977) as well as of CTMM (Resjö et al., 1978; Scotti et al., 1980).

In our series of 110 children examined with CTMM because of dysraphism, we found diastematomyelia in 31 cases (28%), a very high frequency compared with previous reports. As reported by Scotti et al. (1980), a bony spur or bridge or a fibrous septum separating the two parts of the cord is not as common as previously thought and in our material this was seen only in 10 cases (33%) (Fig. 4.11). In all cases with a bony spur or cartilagenous or fibrous septum there was a complete dural sac on each side of the division.

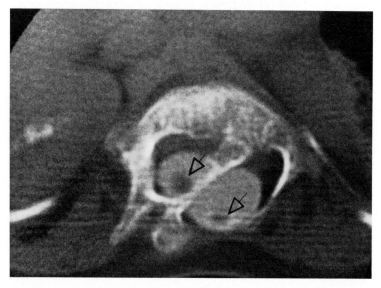

Fig. 4.11. Diastematomyelia. Girl, 5 years, T12. A bony spur divides the spinal canal into two compartments and in each of these there is a dural sac containing one part of the cord (*arrows*).

In the remaining cases (67%) the two parts of the cord were situated in the same dural sac, the extension of the splitting varying between 1 and 11 vertebral levels. The two parts of the cord often appeared slightly asymmetric with a varying degree of separation. Thus there might be an incomplete separation, with strands of neural tissue between the two parts of the cord (Fig. 4.12) or the two parts might be widely separated in the same dural sac (Fig. 4.13). With high resolution CT the nerve roots are clearly visualized emerging from the lateral side of each part of the cord (Fig. 4.12). The CT examinations have also revealed that one or both parts of a split cord is tethered in a much higher frequency than previously reported. In our material this was seen in 21 (68%) of the 31 cases. The diastematomyelia is also often accompanied by other abnormalities of the cord and meninges, such as myelo-meningocele or syringohydromyelia.

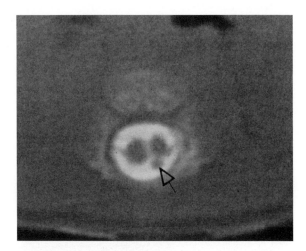

Fig. 4.12. Diastematomyelia and low cord. Girl, 1 month, L3. The two parts of the low cord are connected with strands of neural tissue. From each half there are emerging nerve roots. Posteriorly there is a small amount of lipomatous tissue (*arrow*).

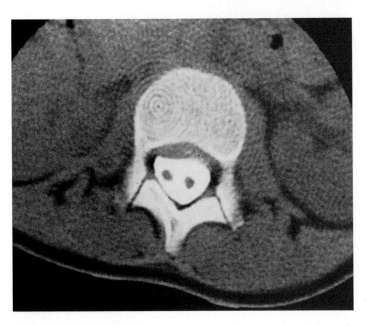

Fig. 4.13. Diastematomyelia. Girl, 10 years, L1. The two halves of the cord are thin and asymmetrically placed in the same dural sac.

Neurenteric Cyst

The neurenteric cyst represents a persistence of the transient open passage (the neurenteric canal of Kovalevsky) at the third embryonic week between the yolk sac and the notochordal canal. The persistence of the canal of Kovalevsky is *always* accompanied by some form of *anterior* vertebral dysraphism as well as abnormalities of neural elements and of tissue derived from the entoderm, for instance, enteric duplications (Harwood-Nash and Fitz, 1976). The neurenteric cyst is most often situated in the upper thoracic region but may occur at any level of the canal.

The lesion was previously regarded as very rare but again with improving neuroradiologic techniques and especially with the introduction of CTMM, the possibility of revealing the lesion has increased (Harwood-Nash and Fitz, 1980). In our series of 110 cases of dysraphism examined with CTMM, we have seen 3 cases of neurenteric cyst. The dysraphism of the anterior vertebral body, the canal of Kovalevsky, and the connection between the canal and the enteric cyst is clearly demonstrated, especially if a high resolution technique is used (Fig. 4.14).

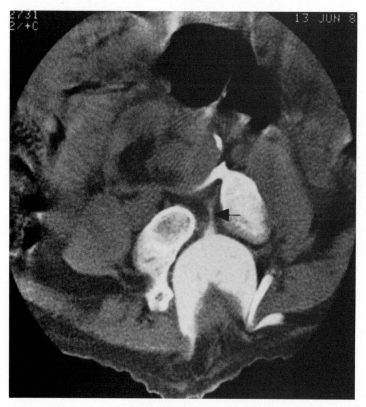

Fig. 4.14. Neurenteric cyst. Boy, 6 years, L5. In a pronounced case of dysraphism, the canal of Kovalevsky is open and a subarachnoid tract is filled with Metrizamide (*arrow*), which enters a small enteric cyst (same case in Fig. 4.5).

Developmental Mass Lesions

Sequestration and overgrowth of normal tissue elements during the embryonic and fetal development of the spinal canal will result in a developmental mass lesion. These lesions may present as the only pathologic change, or may be a part of the wide variety of other dysraphic abnormalities.

Dermoid

The dermoid is derived from epithelium and dermis and may include hair follicles, sebaceous and sweat glands. The epidermoid is derived from epithelium alone. These tumors can be distinguished only histologically and will be treated below as one entity. They may be isolated within the cord, most often in the conus or upper part of the filum terminale, or within the dural sac outside the cord, or in the extradural space. The lumbar region is the most common site, the thoracic region being less often involved, and the cervical region seldom (Harwood-Nash and Fitz, 1976).

At CTMM the tumor may be differentiated from a lipoma because of the differing attenuation values. Depending on the amount of fatty acids contained by the dermoid, the attenuation value of a dermoid may vary between about +30 and −30 Hounsfield units, while a lipoma has considerably lower attenuation, about −60. The examination may also clearly outline a dermal sinus (Fig. 4.15).

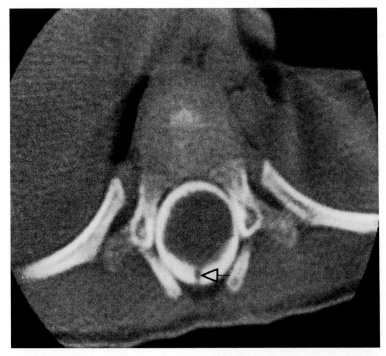

Fig. 4.15. Dermoid. Girl, 5 years, T11. The large intramedullary mass lesion had an attenuation of −20 Hounsfield units. This, combined with a dermal sinus (*arrow*) differentiates the lesion from other tumors.

Teratoma

Teratomas containing derivatives from mesoderm, entoderm, and ectoderm are rarely seen as intraspinal mass lesions (Harwood-Nash and Fitz, 1976). Unlike the dermoids, they present at an early age, mostly before the age of 2 years, and as stated above the teratoma is one of the mass lesions that may involve the entire

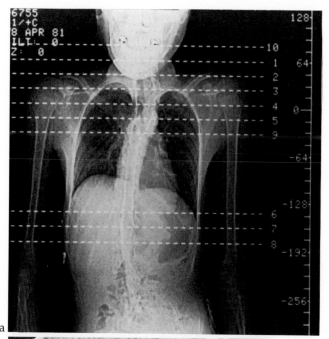

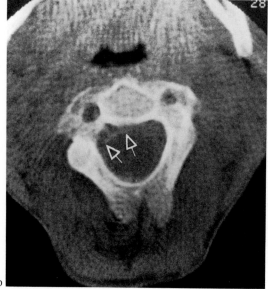

Fig. 4.16. Teratoma. Boy, 17 years.
(a) The Scout view shows an expansile lesion that occupies the entire cord.
(b) In the cervical region (section 1) the lesion almost totally compresses the subarachnoid space, only a small amount of Metrizamide being visible (*arrows*).
(c) In the thoracic region (section 5) the lesion occupies the whole cord and thecal sac. the thin subarachnoid space is filled with Metrizamide (*arrow*). The anatomy of the thoracic vertebrae is severely disorganized.
(d) In the lumbar area (section 8) the lesion is smaller (*arrow*). The position of the nerve roots is disorganized.

The tumor had an attenuation of 20–40 Hounsfield units. Radiologically, it is not possible to distinguish between astrocytoma and teratoma, but occurring in a dysraphic spine the mass is more likely to be a teratoma.

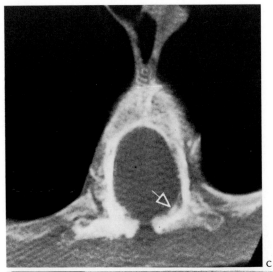

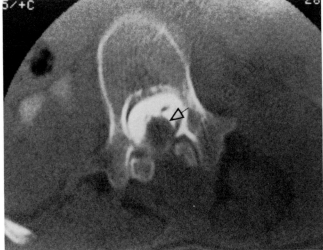

Fig. 4.16. (*Continued*)

cord. At the CTMM they may be difficult to distinguish from dermoids or from neoplastic mass lesions (Fig. 4.16). Sacrococcygeal teratomas, although not considered to be mass lesions of the spinal canal, may be seen together with spinal dysraphism.

Lipoma

As mentioned earlier in this chapter, we consider a lipoma to be a circumscribed mass lesion which should be differentiated from the lipomatous tissue commonly associated with dysraphism. At CTMM the nature of the lesion is revealed by its low attenuation values (about −60 Hounsfield units) (Fig. 4.17).

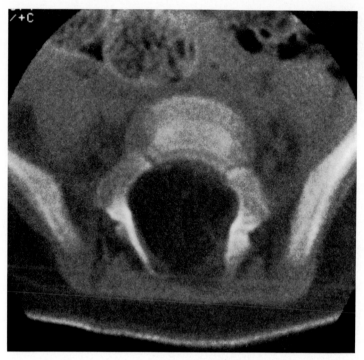

Fig. 4.17. Lipoma. Girl, 9 months, L5. Same patient as in Fig. 2.10. A large lipoma occupies the spinal canal in the lower lumbar and sacral region. Direct coronal section through the tumor (Fig. 2.10) gives the extension of the tumor, and also shows that there is a low cord attached to the lipoma.

Arachnoid Cyst

An arachnoid cyst of the spinal canal may be associated with dysraphism, but may also occur in association with neurofibromatosis or may be acquired due to arachnoiditis. The cyst may be intradural or herniated through the dural into the extradural or even the paravertebral space. The CTMM would reveal a cystic lesion within the intradural sac, or a large noncommunicating cyst outside the dural sac.

Chiari Malformation

The Chiari malformation is a congenital abnormality of the lower brain stem and cerebellum, usually associated with myelomeningocele, or with other manifestations of dysraphism, for instance syringohydromyelia or diastematomyelia (Harwood-Nash and Fitz, 1976). The primary myelographic sign of Chiari malformation is tonsillar herniation. Previously, with conventional myelography, the Chiari malformation might be difficult to distinguish from a craniocervical junction mass due to another cause. However, the CTMM examination of the occipitocervical junction clearly delineates the cord and the herniated tonsils in cases of Chiari malformation (Fig. 4.18). To assess the existence of a Chiari

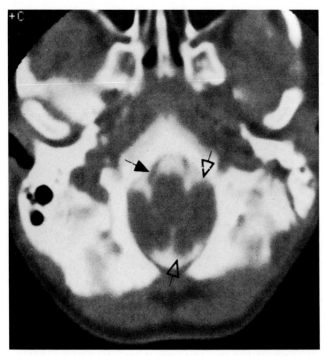

Fig. 4.18. Chiari malformation. Boy, 10 years. The cerebellar tonsils are herniated bilaterally through the foramen magnum (*open arrows*). The medulla is displaced anteriorly and compressed from side to side. On both sides, anteriorly to the medulla, are the vertebral arteries (*black arrow*).

malformation CT sections should be performed at the occipitocervical junction in all CTMMs in cases of dysraphism.

The Complexity of the Dysraphic State

In this chapter, the abnormalities occurring in dysraphism have been described separately. However, the catastrophe occurring in fetal life that causes the dysraphism may to a varying degree involve tissues from ectoderm, entoderm, and mesoderm, and thus a wide spectrum of abnormalities and combinations thereof may occur. The dysraphic anomalies are often associated with sclerotome abnormalities such as deformed ribs, and may be accompanied by cardiopulmonary and/or gastrointestinal anomalies (Harwood-Nash and Fitz, 1976). Also the combination of abnormalities occurring in the tissues derived from the notochord are manifold. This complexity is illustrated in Table 4.1, which describes the changes and combinations of changes seen in 110 CTMMs performed in patients with spinal dysraphism. Usually neonates with obvious meningocele or myelomeningocele will not have myelography at our institution unless there is any specific clinical indication at birth or at a later age. Thus the true frequency of myelomeningocele and its combinations with other abnormalities is higher than shown in the table. Scoliosis caused by vertebral dysraphism occurred in 40% of the cases and spinal stenosis was seen in two cases.

Table 4.1. Abnormalities of the spinal column and canal revealed at CTMM in 110 cases of dysraphism. All figures denote percentage

A. Vertebral dysraphism only	10

B. Widened dural sac and widened dural canal only	2

C. Varying degree of *vertebral dysraphism* and *widening of the dural sac, combined with the following abnormalities* or combinations thereof — 88

	c1	c2	c3	c4	c5	c6	c7	c8	c9	c10	c11	c12	c13	c14	c15	c16	c17	c18	c19	c20	c21	c22	c23	%
Tethered cord, thick filum	×						×	×	×	×	×			×	×	×	×				×	×		(56)
Myelomeningocele	×								×			×	×						×	×	×	×	×	(28)
Lipomatous tissue						×			×			×	×						×	×	×	×	×	(35)
Syringohydromyelia				×			×							×					×		×		×	(21)
Diastematomyelia					×		×				×			×	×	×	×		×		×	×		(28)
Neurenteric cyst			×																			×		(3)
Dermoid				×																				(2)
Teratoma																						×		(1)
Lipoma						×								×					×					(4)
Arachnoid cyst					×																			(1)
Chiari malformation													×				×	×				×		(15)
% of total (n = 110)	8	4	4	2	2	2	13	4	12	2	1	2	2	6	4	1	2	2	3	1	2	8	1	(88)

References

Dale AJD (1969) Diastmatomyelia. Arch Neurol 20: 309–317

Ethier R, King DG, Melancon D, Bélanger G, Taylor S, Thompson C (1979) Development of high resolution computed tomography of the spinal cord. J Comput Assist Tomogr 3: 433–438

Ethier R, King DG, Melancon D, Bélanger G, Thompson C (1980) Diagnosis of intra and extra-medullary lesions by CT without contrast achieved through modifications applied to the EMI CT 5005 body scanner. In: Post MJD (ed) Radiographic evaluation of the spine. Masson, New York, pp 377–393

Fitz CR, Harwood-Nash DC (1975) The tethered conus. AJR 125: 515–523

Forbes WSC, Isherwood I (1978) Computed tomography in syringomyelia and the associated Arnold–Chiari Type I malformation. Neuroradiology 15: 73–78

Gardner WJ (1965) Hydrodynamic mechanism of syringomyelia: its relationship to myelocele. Neurol Neurosurg Psychiatr 28: 247–259

Harwood-Nash DC, Fitz CR (1976) Neuroradiology in infants and children. CV Mosby, St. Louis

Harwood-Nash DC, Fitz CR (1980) Computed tomography and the pediatric spine: computed tomographic Metrizamide myelography in children. In: Post MJD (ed) Radiographic evaluation of the spine. Masson, New York, pp 4–33

Hoffman HJ, Hendrick EB, Humphreys RP (1976) The tethered spinal cord: its protean manifestations, diagnosis and surgical correction. Childs Brain 2: 145–155

James HE, Oliff M (1977) Computed tomography in spinal dysraphism. J Comput Assist Tomogr 1:391–397

Lichtenstein BW (1940) "Spinal dysraphism", spina bifida and myelodysplasia. Arch Neurol Psychiatr 44: 792–810

Lohkampf F, Clausen C, Schumacher G (1978) CT demonstration of pathologic changes of the spinal cord accompanying spina bifida and diastematomyelia. In: Kaufmann HJ (ed) Progress in pediatric radiology. S. Karger, Basel, 5:II, pp 200–227

McRae DL, Standen J (1966) Roentgenologic findings in syringomyelia and hydromyelia. AJR 98: 695–703

Pettersson H, Fitz CR, Harwood-Nash DC, Chuang S, Armstrong E (1982) Adverse effects to myelography with Metrizamide in infants, children and adolescents. II. Local damage caused by the lumbar puncture and contrast medium injection. Acta Radiol [Diagn] (Stockh) in press

Resjö IM, Harwood-Nash DC, Fitz CR, Chuang S (1978) Computed tomographic Metrizamide myelography in spinal dysraphism in infants and children. J Comput Assist Tomogr 2: 549–558

Resjö IM, Harwood-Nash DC, Fitz CR, Chuang S (1979) Computed tomographic Metrizamide myelography in syringohydromyelia. Radiology 131: 405–407

Scotti G, Musgrave MA, Harwood-Nash DC, Fitz CR, Chuang S (1980) Diastematomyelia in children: Metrizamide and CT Metrizamide myelography. AJNR 1: 403–410

Tadmor R, Davis KR, Roberson GH, Chapman PH (1977) The diagnosis of diastematomyelia by computed tomography. Surg Neurol 8: 434–436

Weinstein MA, Rothner AD, Duchesneau P, Dohn DF (1975) Computed tomography in diastematomyelia. Radiology 117: 609–611

Wickbom IW, Hanafee W (1963) Soft tissue masses immediately below the foramen magnum. Acta Radiol [Diagn] (Stockh) 1: 647–658

Wolpert SM, Scott RM, Carter BL (1977) Computed tomography in spinal dyraphism. Surg Neurol 8: 199–06

Chapter 5
Neoplasms

Mass lesions within the spinal canal, or lesions in the spinal column or the paravertebral space with extension into the canal are not common in children. Early clinical signs of an intraspinal mass lesion in a child may be subtle and radiographic abnormalities revealed at plain film X-ray may often be absent. Because of this, intraspinal neoplasms and neoplasms of the vertebrae or the paravertebral space are often quite large before they come to sophisticated neuroradiologic examinations.

Primary neoplasms of neural origin, such as astrocytoma, ependymoma, and neurofibroma, may develop within the cord, nerve roots, and meninges. Others, such as neuroblastoma-ganglioneuroma, may also develop within paraspinal nervous tissue, the tumor extending into the spinal canal.

Primary neoplasms of the spine, as well as those of para-spinal structures other than nervous tissue, e.g., retroperitoneal sarcomas, may extend directly into the spinal canal; this may also occur with pelvic tumors.

Metastases to the spinal canal may be CSF borne from primary tumors elsewhere in the CNS, or they may be blood borne, e.g., lymphomas or leukemic infiltrations. Metastatic lesions in the vertebrae may extend directly into the spinal canal in the same way as primary tumors of the spinal column.

The neoplasms may be situated within the spinal cord (intramedullary), within the dura but outside the cord (extramedullary, intradural), or in the extradural space. They may also occupy two or three of these compartments, although this is uncommon in children (Harwood-Nash and Fitz, 1980). With conventional examinations, including oil or Metrizamide myelography, it might be difficult to localize the lesion concerning its position vis-à-vis the dura and the cord. The CTMM, giving fine anatomic detail, and providing transaxial sections through the cord and dura, has increased diagnostic accuracy concerning localization in this respect. It also provides information on the composition of the tumor, not possible to obtain by conventional radiographic examinations.

Primary Neoplasms of Neural Origin

Primary malignant neoplasms of neural origin are rare, with an annual incidence rate in the United States of about three per million (calculated from Young and Miller [1975] in their report of the Third National Cancer Survey, and the assumption that 10% of all CNS malignancies in childhood occur in the spine [Harwood-Nash and Fitz, 1980]).

Neurofibroma, a histologically benign tumor of neural origin, is also rare in absolute figures but among the neoplasms of neural origin it is common according to the Mayo series reported by Sloof et al. (1964), occurring in 29% of all intraspinal neoplasms at all ages.

The tumors of the group denoted as neuroblastoma-ganglioneuroma are more common in children, with an annual incidence of about 8 in a million (Young and Miller, 1975).

Astrocytoma

Astrocytoma, although uncommon, is the most frequent glioma of the cord in children. In a large series of intraspinal neoplasms earlier reported from this institution, astrocytomas constituted 8% of intraspinal mass lesions (Harwood-Nash and Fitz, 1976). The lesions are most often situated in the cervical region, involving several vertebral segments, but may even involve the majority of the cord. They may grow very slowly, and they may even involve the entire cord before they give symptoms pronounced enough to indicate a thorough neuroradiologic examination.

The CTMM examination reveals a large intramedullary tumor, often with irregular margins and partially adherent to the dura (Fig. 5.1). The astrocytoma may be cystic or solid, which might be differentiated by the differing attenuation values. A pronounced vascularization of the tumor may be revealed by enhancement after intravenous contrast medium injection (Handel et al., 1978).

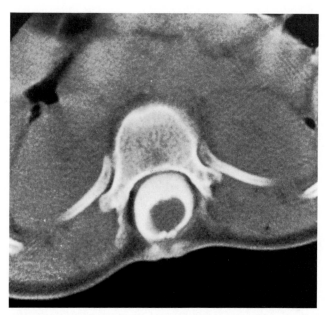

Fig. 5.1. Astrocytoma. Girl, 8 years, T12. The cord is irregularly enlarged. The attenuation value is 20 Hounsfield units. As the tumor appeared in a patient with dysraphism, the differentiation between astrocytoma, ependymoma, and dermoid is difficult.

Ependymoma

Ependymoma, comprising 6% of all intraspinal mass lesions in the series from The Hospital for Sick Children, Toronto (Harwood-Nash and Fitz, 1976), arise from ependymal cells in the cord or filum terminale. The lumbar region is most commonly involved, although in rare cases, the tumor may extend up into the thoracic area. Cervical involvement is extremely rare. From a radiographic point of view we consider only the ependymoma of the filum terminale alone to be extramedullary.

At the CTMM examination the tumor appears as a gentle widening of the cord or filum terminale (Fig. 5.2), or as a more abrupt and eccentric nodular extension. As in the astrocytoma, the ependymoma might be cystic or solid, and the differential diagnosis at CTMM between an intramedullary astrocytoma, ependymoma, dermoid, or teratoma, and syringohydromyelia with closed obex may be very difficult.

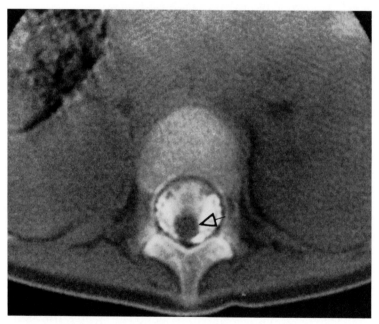

Fig. 5.2. Ependymoma of the filum terminale. Girl, 1 year, T12. The filum is smoothly enlarged (*arrow*). The nerve roots are displaced anteriorly and laterally.

Neurofibroma, Neurofibrosarcoma

A neurofibroma is composed of cells derived from the nerve sheath, probably the Schwann cells. It may appear as a solitary tumor or as multiple neurofibromas or a large plexiform tumor in Von Recklinghausen's disease. The tumor may be situated in the intradural compartment, or in the extradural, or both. We have had two cases of neurofibromatosis, and both were extradural (Fig. 5.3).

The spectrum of other radiologic changes occurring in and around the spinal column in Von Recklinghausen's disease will be discussed in Chap. 7.

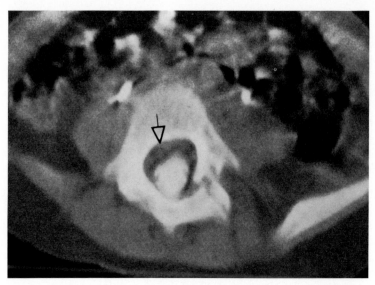

Fig. 5.3. Neurofibroma. Boy, 8 years, L5. The extradural mass in the anterior part of the spinal canal (*arrow*) displaces the dural sac dorsally, with a slight impression in the sac. Note also the dysplastic vertebra.

Neuroblastoma, Ganglioneuroma

The tumors of the group denoted as neuroblastoma-ganglioneuroma arise from the adrenal gland or the sympathetic chain extending from the base of the skull to the pelvis. There are no distinct borders between the different types of the tumors included in this group, and there might be spontaneous tumor regression from the more malignant neuroblastoma to the more benign ganglioneuroblastoma and ganglioneuroma (Bolande, 1971).

Intraspinal involvement of the tumor is seen in a frequency that ranges between 14% and 17% according to different authors (Armstrong et al., 1982; King et al., 1975; Traggis et al., 1977). Calcification of the tumor occurs in about 25% of all chest and abdominal lesions, but is very seldom seen in the intraspinal part of the tumor (Armstrong et al., 1982; Prakach, 1969).

Our experience with CT examination of this lesion emanates from the 77 patients whose tumors were diagnosed at our hospital in the period 1976–80 (Armstrong et al., 1981). Of these patients, 58 had a CT examination, and 18 of these also a CTMM. Of these 18 patients, 11 had intraspinal extension of the tumor, and this was unexpected from a clinical point of view in 6. It is important for the surgeon to know preoperatively if there is any intraspinal extension, as this knowledge will determine the surgical approach and/or the radiotheraphy. Futhermore, if a neuroblastoma is operated on without the knowledge of intraspinal extension, there is a risk of intraspinal hemorrhage and damage to the cord.

We have found that primary CTMM is the method of choice in the examination of patients with neuroblastoma-ganglioneuroma as it will give information on both the extra- and intraspinal part of the tumor. CTMM, combined with intravenous contrast medium injection, will give more information than any other imaging modality concerning the site and composition of the primary tumor and of metastases, as well as of intraspinal extension.

The extension of the tumor from the paravertebral to the intraspinal space may be seen at the CTMM examination as widening of the intervertebral foramina. This is seen at the conventional plain radiograph too, but the CTMM also shows the tumor in the widened foramen (Fig. 5.4). Tumor growth within the spinal canal may displace the cord and dural sac without any compression of these structures (Fig. 5.5). This displacement, no matter how slight, is sufficient for diagnosis,

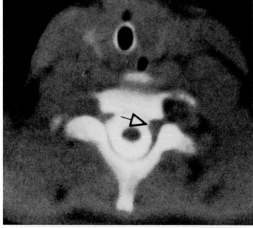

Fig. 5.4. Ganglioneuroma. Girl, 6 years, C6. The extraspinal part of the tumor in the neck continues through the widened intervertebral foramen and invades the intraspinal space where it impinges on the sac (*arrow*).

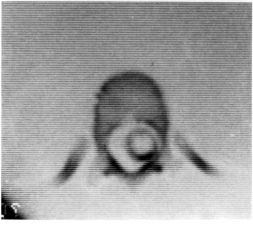

Fig. 5.5. Neuroblastoma. Girl, 13 years, T11. Tumor growth in the spinal canal, displacing but not deforming the dural sac.

especially in the thoracic spine, where the epidural space is constantly symmetric, provided there is no scoliosis. The tumor may also flatten one side of the dural sac (Fig. 5.6), or impinge on the sac (Fig. 5.4). In pronounced cases there might be a complete block for the contrast medium passage. It should be noted that intraspinal extension of the tumor may not correspond to the paraspinal part but extend several vertebral levels cranial or caudal from the paraspinal tumor, and the clinical signs are often minimal.

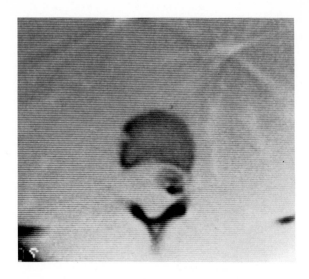

Fig. 5.6. Neuroblastoma. Same patient as in Fig. 5.5, L1. Pronounced intraspinal tumor growth displaces and deforms the dural sac. No neurologic abnormalities were present.

Primary Neoplasms of the Spinal Column and Paraspinal Structures

Primary tumors of the spine with direct extension to the spinal canal are very rare (Harwood-Nash and Fitz, 1976) and no incidence rates can be given. At the CT examination it may be difficult to distinguish between malignant lesions such as Ewing's sarcoma, osteogenic sarcoma, or rhabdomyosarcoma and benign lesions such as hemangioma and giant cell tumors. They all give a mottled appearance with multiple osteolytic areas (Fig. 5.7), often enhancing following intravenous contrast medium injection (Harwood-Nash and Fitz, 1980). More often than not, these tumors are confined to the vertebral body, not impinging on the spinal canal. Osteoblastomas, often situated in the pedicles and laminae of a cervical vertebra, and aneurysmal bone cysts, may both compromise the spinal canal to a considerable degree (Bonakdarpour et al., 1978; McLeod et al., 1976) well detectable at CTMM (Figs. 5.8. 5.9).

Histiocytosis X, although a generalized disease of the reticulo-endothelial system, may present itself as a localized osteolytic lesion in one vertebra. The vertebral body involved may be compressed and the disease may spread into the epidural space and impinge on the cord. This is clearly visualized at the CTMM (Fig. 5.10). However, the skeletal lesion may to a high degree mimic, for instance, Ewing's sarcoma, and radiologic differentiation may be difficult or impossible, whatever imaging modality is used.

Paraspinal malignancies may spread to the extradural space by direct intrusion, the most common being retroperitoneal sarcoma, teratoma, or neuroblastoma in the small child, and neurofibrosarcoma and ganglioneuroma in the older child. The advantage of CTMM in the examination of neuroblastoma-ganglioneuroma has been described above. CTMM has proved to be a very valuable tool in the examination of other paraspinal tumors, especially in the pelvis. The CT examination shows the extension of the tumor within the bone itself, its extension into the spinal canal, and also demonstrates the soft tissue mass and its effect upon the

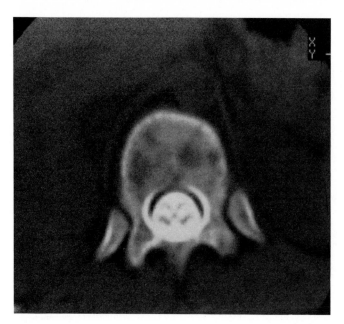

Fig. 5.7. Ewing's sarcoma. Boy, 14 years, T12. The neoplasm has a mottled appearance with multiple osteolytic areas.

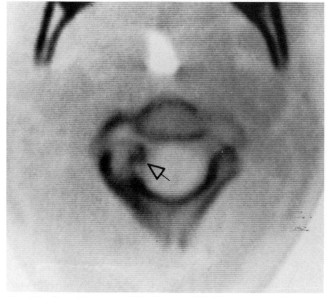

Fig. 5.8. Osteoblastoma. Girl, 11 years, C5. The tumor impinges on the spinal canal (*arrow*) and the right transversal foramen.

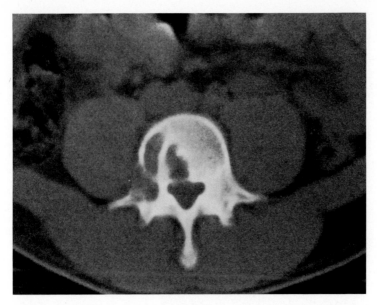

Fig. 5.9. Aneurysmal bone cyst. Boy, 7 years, L4. This tumor expands the vertebral body, and impinges upon the spinal canal anteriorly and the intervertebral foramen.

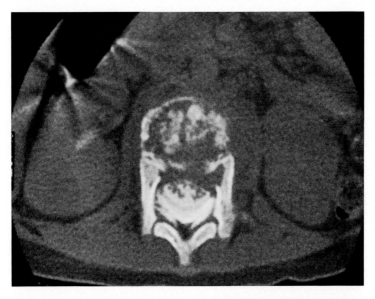

Fig. 5.10. Histiocytosis X. Boy, 3 years, L2. Pronounced osteolytic destruction of the vertebra with tumor growth into the spinal canal, compressing the dural sac and cauda equina. There is a considerable leakage of Metrizamide in the extradural space dorsal to the sac.

intra-abdominal structures (Berger and Kuhn, 1978; Harwood-Nash and Fitz, 1980; Nakagawa et al., 1977; Reilly, 1977). CT has also proved to be particularly valuable in the follow-up of nonoperative therapy of these tumors.

Metastases

CSF-borne metastases from neoplasms elsewhere in the CNS are the most common secondary tumors of the spinal canal (Harwood-Nash and Fitz, 1976). Intracranial medulloblastoma in particular (McFarland et al., 1969), ependymomas (Svien et al., 1949), astrocytomas, pineal neoplasms, and carcinoma of the choroid plexus (Harwood-Nash and Fitz, 1976) are the primary tumors most often involved. The CTMM reveals multiple nodules around the nerve roots and in the cauda equina, and sheathing around the cord, which may appear enlarged, with irregular margins (Resjö et al., 1979) (Fig. 5.11).

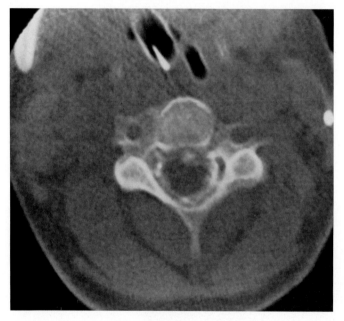

Fig. 5.11. Metastatic pineal dysgerminoma. Girl, 12 years, C3. The cervical cord appears irregularly enlarged because of sheathing of tumor around the cord.

Lymphoma and leukemia may spread to the intra- or extradural space (Bharati and Kalyanaraman, 1973; Wilhyde et al., 1963). The CTMM appearance of this spread will be an extradural mass, or multiple nodules along the cord and along the nerve roots of the cauda equina (Fig. 5.12). The irregular enlargement of the nerve roots caused by these nodules should be differentiated from the smoother enlargement of the nerve roots seen in Déjerine–Sotta's disease, which is an uncommon hypertrophic interstitial neuropathy (Harwood-Nash and Fitz, 1976; Rao et al., 1974).

Metastases to the vertebrae from distant primary tumors are rare in children, the one most often seen being rhabdomyosarcoma (Harwood-Nash and Fitz, 1976). These metastases may be large, destroying the vertebral body and extending para- and intraspinally (Fig. 5.13)

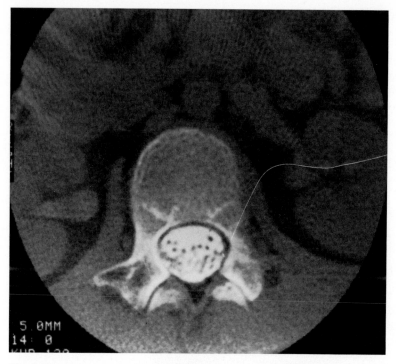

Fig. 5.12

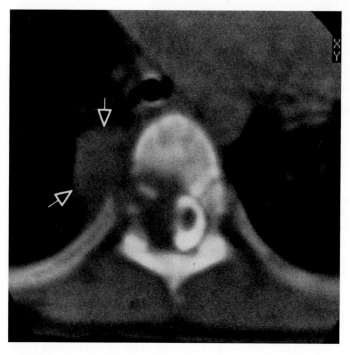

Fig. 5.13

Enhancement of Lesions After Intravenous Contrast Medium Injection

Although of much less importance than in CT of the brain, the intravenous contrast medium injection may add information also in CTMM. This is especially valid where mass lesions are concerned, and therefore will be briefly discussed here.

There have been isolated reports of chemical detection of iodine in the CSF after intravenous contrast medium injection (Lampe et al., 1970; McLennan and Becker, 1971). Coin et al. (1979) reported on enhancement of the CSF in the spinal subarachnoid space detectable at CT examination. However, this enhancement did not allow any detailed studies of the intraspinal structures. Direct enhancement of the cord, detectable at CT examination, has been reported by Isherwood et al. (1977) and Resjö et al. (1979). As mentioned in Chap. 2, the normal cord may enhance slightly after intravenous contrast medium injection, with an increase of the attenuation value of about 10 Hounsfield units.

Highly vascularized tumors may enhance considerably. Nakagawa et al. (1977) first described enhancement of a hemangioblastoma and we have had one case of a widespread hemangioma, in which both the paraspinal and intraspinal part enhanced to about 100 Hounsfield units after contrast medium injection (Fig. 5.14). We have also had one case of intraspinal arteriovenous malformation that enhanced considerably after intravenous contrast medium injection (Fig. 5.15). Also a highly vascular astrocytoma might enhance after intravenous contrast medium injection (Handel et al., 1978).

Malignant lesions of the vertebral bodies may be highly vascularized and show marked enhancement, and in CT examination of paraspinal lesions with intraspinal extension, as for instance neuroblastoma-ganglioneuroma, CTMM combined with intravenous contrast medium injection is of great value (Armstrong et al., 1982; Harwood-Nash and Fitz, 1980).

Recently we have also shown that there may be a pronounced enhancement of the spinal cord and roots in children who have had therapeutic irradiation of paraspinal tumors, the radiation field including the cord (Pettersson et al., 1981). Probably this represents a subclinical myelitis induced by the radiation.

The value of intravenous contrast medium injection as a complement to the CTMM will probably increase in the future, with increasing spatial resolution and contrast discrimination provided by the CT equipment.

◁ **Fig. 5.12.** Leukemic infiltration. Boy, 9 years, L2. Nodules of leukemic tissue on the nerve roots of the cauda equina create an appearance of an increased number of roots, and the normal symmetry is disturbed.

◁ **Fig. 5.13.** Metastatic rhabdomyosarcoma. Boy, 4 years, T2. The paraspinal part of the metastasis is clearly visible (*arrows*) as is the destruction of the vertebra and the intraspinal invasion. The dural sac is dislocated and compressed, as is the cord.

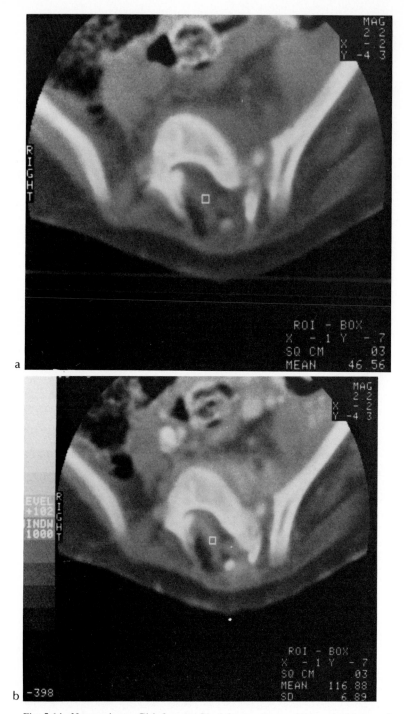

Fig. 5.14. Hemangioma. Girl, 2 years, S1. A large extra- and intraspinal hemangioma in a patient with dysraphism (a) before, and (b) after intravenous contrast medium injection. The intraspinal part of the hemangioma enhances from an attenuation of 46 to an attenuation of 116 Hounsfield units (as measured within the white square).

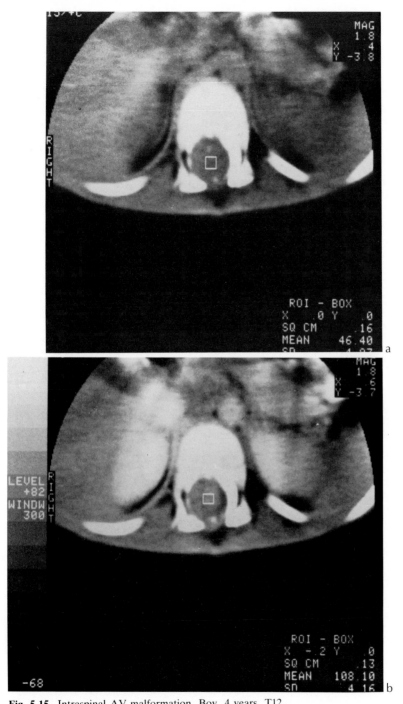

Fig. 5.15. Intraspinal AV malformation. Boy, 4 years, T12.
(a) Before contrast medium injection. The AV malformation presents as a large intramedullary mass compressing the Metrizamide-filled subarachnoid space. Note the calcifications of phleboliths within the mass.
(b) After intravenous contrast medium injection. There is a pronounced enhancement of the tumor, with an attenuation value increasing from 46 to 108 Hounsfield units.

References

Armstrong E, Harwood-Nash DC, Fitz CR, Chuang S, Pettersson H, Martin DJ (1982) Computed
    tomography of the neuroblastoma-ganglioneuroma spectrum in children. AJR, in press
Berger PE, Kuhn JP (1978) Computed tomography of tumours of the musculoskeletal system in
    children. Clinical applications. Radiology 127: 171–175
Bharati RS, Kalyanaraman S (1973) Epidural spinal lymphoma in an infant. J Neurosurg 39: 412–415
Bolande RP (1971) Benignity of neonatal tumours and concept of cancer repression in early life. Am J
    Dis Child 122: 12–14
Bonakdarpour A, Levy WM, Aegerter E (1978) Primary and secondary aneurysmal bone cyst: a
    radiological study of 75 cases. Radiology 126: 75–83
Coin CG, Keranen VJ, Pennink M, Ahmad WD (1979) Evidence of CSF enhancement in the spinal
    subarachnoid space after intravenous contrast medium administration: is intravenous computer
    assisted myelography possible? J Comput Assist Tomogr 3: 267–269
Handel S, Grossman R, Sarwar M (1978) Computed tomography in the diagnosis of spinal cord
    astrocytoma. J Comput Assist Tomogr 2: 226–228
Harwood-Nash DC, Fitz CR (1976) Neuroradiology in infants and children. CV Mosby, St. Louis
Harwood-Nash DC, Fitz CR (1980) Computed tomography and the pediatric spine: computed
    tomographic Metrizamide myelography in children. In: Post MJD (ed) Radiographic evaluation of
    the spine. Masson, New York, pp 4–33
Isherwood I, Fawcitt RA, Nettle JR, Spencer JW, Pullan BR (1977) Computer tomography of the
    spine. A preliminary report. In: du Boulay GH, Moseley IF (eds). Computerized axial tomography
    in clinical practice. Springer-Verlag, Berlin-Heidelberg-New York, pp 322–335
King D, Goodman J, Hawk T, Boles ET, Sayers MP (1975) Dumbbell neuroblastomas in children. Arch
    Surg 110: 888–891
Lampe KF, James G, Erbesfield M, Mende TJ, Viamonte M (1970) Cerebrovascular permeability of a
    water-soluble contrast material, Hypaque (sodium diatrizoate). Experimental study in dogs. Invest
    Radiol 5: 79–85
McClennan BL, Becker JA (1971) Cerebrospinal fluid transfer of contrast material at urography. AJR
    113: 427–432
McFarland DR, Horwitz H, Saenger EL, Bahr GK (1969) Medulloblastoma—a review of prognosis and
    survival. Br J Radiol 42: 198–214
McLeod RA, Dahlin DC, Beabout JW (1976) The spectrum of osteoblastoma. AJR 126: 321–335
Nakagawa H, Huang YP, Malis LI, Wolf BS (1977) Computed tomography of intraspinal and paraspinal
    neoplasms. J Comput Assist Tomogr 1: 377–390
Pettersson H, Harwood-Nash DC, Fitz CR, Chuang S, Armstrong E (1981) Computed tomographic
    intravenous myelography of the irradiated cord in children. AJNR 2: 581–584
Prakach B (1969) Neuroblastoma and ganglioneuroblastoma causing spinal cord compression. J Oslo
    City Hospital 19: 200–210
Rao CV, Fitz CR, Harwood-Nash DC (1974) Déjerine–Sotta's syndrome in children. AJR 122: 70–74
Reilly BJ (1977) Extracranial computerized tomography in children. Comput Tomogr 1: 257–270
Resjö IM, Harwood-Nash DC, Fitz CR, Chuang S (1979) CT Metrizamide myelography for intraspinal
    and paraspinal neoplasms in infants and children. AJR 132: 367–372
Resjö IM, Harwood-Nash DC, Fitz CR, Chuang S (1979) Normal cord in infants and children examined
    with computed tomographic Metrizamide myelography. Radiology 130: 691–696
Sloof JL, Kernohan JW, MacCarty CS (1964) Primary intramedullary tumours of the spinal cord and
    filum terminale. WB Saunders, Philadephia
Svien HJ, Gates EM, Kernohan JW (1949) Spinal subarachnoid implantation associated with ependy-
    moma. Arch Neurol Psychiatr 62: 847–856
Traggis DG, Filler RM, Druckman H, Jaffe N, Cassady JR (1977) Prognosis for children with
    neuroblastoma presenting with paralysis. J Pediatr Surg 12: 419–425
Wilhyde DE, Jane JA, Mullan S (1963) Spinal epidural leukemia. Am J Med 34: 281–287
Young JL, Miller RW (1975) Incidence of malignant tumours in US children. J Pediatr 86: 254–258

Chapter 6
Trauma, Infection, and Inflammation

Minor trauma to the spine is common in childhood, but more severe traumatic lesions of the spinal canal with neurologic disturbances are uncommon, accounting for about 5% of the indications for myelography at The Hospital for Sick Children, Toronto. The cause of the lesion is most often birth injuries in neonates, and traffic accidents or falls in older children. Infection of the spinal column and canal is also uncommon in children, accounting for 3% of the myelographies at our hospital. Early and effective treatment of both traumatic and infectious lesions may prevent serious irreparable damage, and thus an accurate diagnostic work-up is urgent. In this respect, the introduction of CT and CTMM has considerably improved the diagnostic sensitivity and specificity of these lesions.

Trauma

The CTMM has proved to be very valuable in the evaluation of patients with spinal trauma. This is partly due to the technique, as Metrizamide may be introduced into the subarachnoid space at the level C1–C2, using the lateral approach, and the entire examination may be performed without changing the patient's supine position (Naidich et al., 1979). The standard radiographs of the spine are superior in evaluation of the overall alteration of the shape and structure of the spine, but the CT examination will demonstrate the subtle fractures, especially at the C1–C2 level (Geehr et al., 1978; Kerschner et al., 1977), as well as the dislocation of the fragments and distortions of the canal (Tadmor, 1978). The information on the skeletal damage achieved by the CT examination is superior to that provided by the conventional tomogram, although conventional tomography in the sagittal plane may still add information to that provided by the CT. The CTMM will also reveal accumulations of blood in the spinal canal, as well as impingement on the cord or dural sac by fracture fragments or hematomas and direct lesions of the cord itself will also be seen. At the same examination fractures of the pelvis, as well as lesions of the chest, abdomen, or pelvic cavity may be assessed.

It is important to obtain CT sections as perpendicular as possible to the axis of each part of the spine. Oblique images may be confusing, especially in the presence of malalignment of vertebral bodies or fragments thereof. As mentioned in Chap. 2, it is now possible to re-form images in the plane perpendicular to the long axis of the spine. Also reconstruction in the sagittal and/or coronal plane often will add important information (Kaiser et al., 1981).

Fractures

Fractures with disruption of the vertebral bodies, common in adults (Naidich, 1979), are rare in children. The transaxial sections reveal fractures through the vertebral bodies and the neural arch (Fig. 6.1) and sagittal reconstruction may demonstrate the posterior fragments emanating from the vertebral body as well as showing if this fragment is compressing the dural sac or cord (Kaiser et al., 1981).

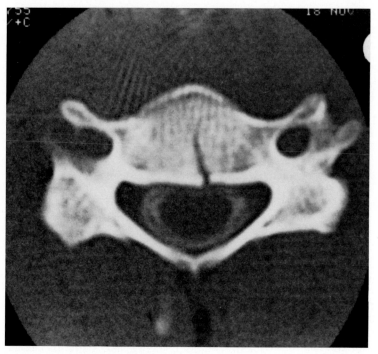

Fig. 6.1. Fracture of the vertebral body. Girl, 14 years, C4. Same case as in Fig. 2.8. A diastatic fracture of C4. Note compression of the Metrizamide-filled subarachnoid space, cord, and nerve roots.

Herniation of Intervertebral Discs

Herniation of the intervertebral discs may occur in adolescence, although rarely (Garrido et al., 1978). In the CTMM it will appear as an extradural mass lesion, possibly impinging on the roots (Coin, 1980; Coin et al., 1977; Harwood-Nash, 1977). In children the herniation is usually large and therefore easily revealed by the CT examination.

Avulsion of the Vertebral Apophysis

Avulsion of the vertebral apophysis and posterior dislocation of its posterior part is very rare, but may occur in adolescence. If the avulsed part is ossified, it may be revealed by conventional radiologic examination including myelography. The CT appearance of this lesion was first described by Handel et al. (1979), and Pettersson et al. (1981) showed that CT examination with sagittal reconstruction will give exact information on the nature of the lesion, as well as its extension in the spinal canal (Fig. 6.2).

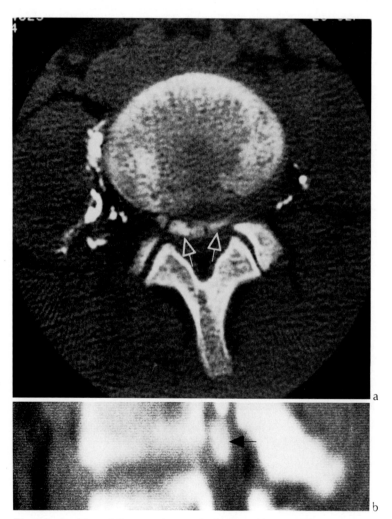

Fig. 6.2. Avulsion of the posterior apophysis. Boy, 14 years, L4.
(a) The fragmented posterior apophysis (*arrows*) is posteriorly dislocated into the spinal canal. At both sides of the vertebra there is Pantopaque, from previous examination performed elsewhere.
(b) the sagittal reconstruction shows that the fragment is dislocated posteriorly and cranially in the canal (*arrow*). The dense area superior to the fragment is Pantopaque.

Spondylolysis and Spondylolisthesis

In spondylolysis and spondylolisthesis the CT examination may clearly reveal the lesion through the neural arch as well as dislocation of the vertebral body (Nakagawa et al., 1980).

Avulsion of the Nerve Roots

Avulsion of the nerve roots and disruption of the meninges may occur in any trauma if violent enough, but in childhood it is most often seen after traumatic deliveries (Harwood-Nash and Fitz, 1976). The tearing often occurs in the low cervical cord which is an area difficult to examine properly by conventional radiographic techniques. However, the lesion may lead to extra-arachnoid CSF leakage, easily revealed by the CTMM (Fig. 6.3).

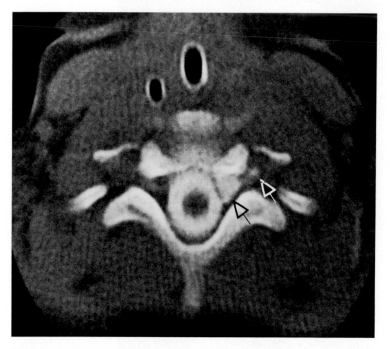

Fig. 6.3. Avulsed nerve root. Girl, 1 year. At the C7 level, there has been an avulsion of a nerve root with disruption of the meninges, and leakage of Metrizamide out through the left intervertebral foramen (*arrows*).

Intramedullary Hematomas

Intramedullary hematomas may be differentiated from edema of the cord by differing attenuation values, and also an extradural hematoma may be revealed by its high Hounsfield numbers (Post, 1980).

Cord Atrophy

Cord atrophy is one sequela of severe injury. It appears as a small asymmetric cord within a normal-sized dural sac (Fig. 6.4). A hemorrhage within the cord may also heal with cyst formation, simulating syringohydromyelia, although often limited to only a few vertebral segments.

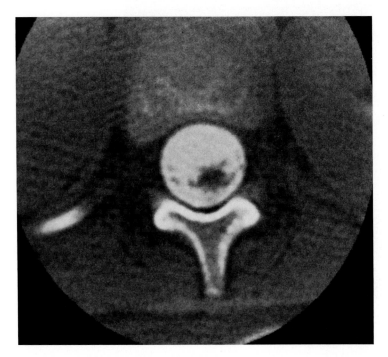

Fig. 6.4. Atrophic cord. Girl, 5 years, T12. There is atrophy of the lower part of the cord at the T12 level as a sequela of a spinal trauma, with ensuing paraplegia. The conus is very small, and asymmetrically placed in the subarachnoid space (cf. normal cord, Fig. 3.11).

Infection and Inflammation

The introduction of CT and CTMM has meant a considerable improvement in the diagnostic accuracy of inflammatory lesions, although the improvement is less pronounced than that concerning trauma. Especially in complicated infections, CTMM may add information to the conventional radiographic methods (Bolivar et al., 1978).

Osteomyelitis

In osteomyelitis the CT appearance, with destruction, new bone formation, and irregular contrast enhancement may be difficult to differentiate from malignant neoplasms and histiocytosis X. However, an extradural abscess may well be imaged by CTMM, as will new bone formation in the healing stage of the disease (Fig. 6.5).

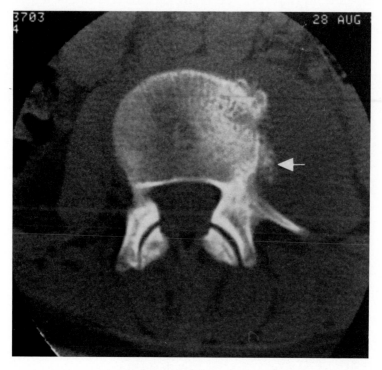

Fig. 6.5. Osteomyelitis. Girl, 15 years, L4. Note the new bone formation (*arrow*) in the healing stage.

Intraspinal Infections

Intraspinal infections may affect the spinal cord and roots, as well as the meninges. Abscess or empyema is most often situated in the extradural space (Harwood-Nash and Fitz, 1976). In the CTMM these abscesses will probably enhance in their peripheries, similarly to brain abscesses. We have no experience of CTMM in intraspinal abscess, and there seem to be no such reports on record.

Transverse Myelitis

Transverse myelitis may uncommonly appear as a non-specific swelling of the cord (Harwood-Nash and Fitz, 1976) (Fig. 6.6), but the cord may as well appear normal at the CTMM, as it will at the conventional myelography.

Arachnoiditis

Arachnoiditis is in our material most often caused by lumboperitoneal shunts. CTMM reveals a pronounced narrowing and irregularity of the subarachnoid

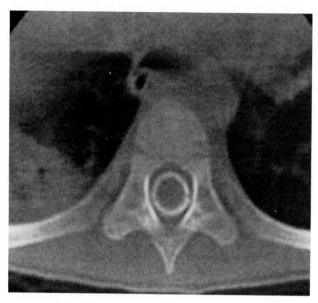

Fig. 6.6. Transverse myelitis. Boy, 3 years, T8. This appears as a nonspecific swelling of the cord (cf. normal cord, Fig. 3.10).

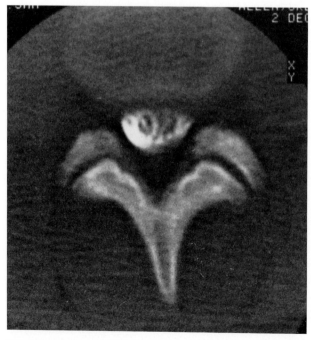

Fig. 6.7. Arachnoiditis. Girl, 17 years, L3. The dural sac is shrunk, and the nerve roots are disorganized and irregularly bunched (cf. normal cauda equina, Fig. 3.14).

space, often over several levels, both in the lumbar, thoracic, and cervical regions (Fig. 6.7). Both in conventional myelography and in CTMM there are considerable similarities in the radiographic appearance of tumor seeding to the cord and roots, arachnoiditis, and Déjerine–Sotta's disease. However, it should be possible to differentiate between the three conditions at the CTMM examination, as the tumor seeding appears in a normal-sized or expanded subarachnoid space, while the arachnoiditis gives an irregular shrinkage of the dural sac. In Déjerine–Sotta's disease, the enlargement of the roots is smoother and more regular than in arachnoiditis or in metastatic disease (Rao et al., 1974).

References

Bolivar R, Kohl S, Pickering LK (1978) Vertebral osteomyelitis in children: report of four cases. Pediatrics 62: 549–553

Coin CG (1980) Computed tomography of the spine. In: Post MJD (ed). Radiographic evaluation of the spine. Masson, New York, pp 394–412

Coin CG, Chan YS, Keranen V, Pennink M (1977) Computer assisted myelography in disk disease. J Comput Assist Tomogr 1: 398–404

Garrido E, Humphreys RP, Hendrick EB, Hoffman HJ (1978) Lumbar disc disease in children. Neurosurgery 2: 22–26

Geehr RB, Rothman SL, Kier EL (1978) The role of computed tomography in the evaluation of upper cervical spine pathology. Comput Tomogr 2: 79–97

Handel SF, Twiford TW Jr, Reigel DH, Kaufman HH (1979) Posterior lumbar apophyseal fractures. Radiology 130: 629–633

Harwood-Nash DC (1977) Computed tomography of the spine. In: Norman D, Korobkin M, Newton TH (eds). Computed tomography. University of California Press, San Francisco, pp 342–352

Harwood-Nash DC, Fitz CR (1976) Neuroradiology in infants and children. CV Mosby, St. Louis

Kaiser MC, Pettersson H, Harwood-Nash DC, Fitz CR, Chuang S (1981) CT in trauma to the skull base and spine in children. Neuroradiology 22: 27–31

Kershner MS, Goodman GA, Perlmutter GS (1977) Computed tomography in the diagnosis of an atlas fracture. AJR 128: 688–689

Naidich TP, Pudlowski RM, Moran CJ, Gilula LA, Murphy W, Naidich JB (1979). Computed tomography of spinal fractures. In: Thompson RA, Green JR (eds). Advances in neurology 22: 207–253

Nakagawa H, Malis LI, Huang YP (1980) Computed tomography of soft tissue masses related to the spinal column. In: Post MJD (ed). Radiographic evaluation of the spine. Masson, New York, pp 320–352

Pettersson H, Harwood-Nash DC, Fitz CR, Chuang S, Armstrong E (1981) The CT appearance of avulsion of the posterior vertebral apophysis: case report. Neuroradiology 21: 145–147

Post MJD (1980) CT update: the impact of time, Metrizamide and high resolution on the diagnosis of spinal pathology. In: Post MJD (ed). Radiographic evaluation of the spine. Masson, New York, pp 259–294

Rao CV, Fitz CR, Harwood-Nash DC (1974) Déjerine–Sotta's syndrome in children. AJR 122: 70–74

Tadmor R, Davis KR, Roberson GH, New PFJ, Taveras JM (1978) Computed tomographic evaluation of traumatic spinal injuries. Radiology 127: 825–827

Chapter 7
Musculoskeletal Disorders and Dysplasias Involving the Spinal Column and Canal

Generalized musculoskeletal disorders and dysplasias with involvement of the spinal column and canal constitute a very complex and heterogeneous group. Neuromuscular disorders may mold the growing spine in a disordered fashion, causing, for example, scoliosis. The disorders may also cause a stenosis of the canal and compression of the cord, or conversely, the spinal canal may be widened with a wide ectatic dural sac. The dysplastic changes may also affect tissues other than muscles and bones, as for instance in neurofibromatosis, in which there is a wide spectrum of abnormalities involving tissues of neuroectodermal and mesodermal origin.

Spinal Stenosis

Spinal stenosis may be developmental, occurring as the only abnormality. This type of stenosis may be widespread, involving all the segments of the canal, or it may be localized only to one or two levels, with or without dysraphism (Verbiest, 1954, 1955). The symptoms often do not appear until late in adolescence or adulthood, when a small and normally insignificant bulging of an intervertebral disc, or a likewise normally insignificant bony or ligamentum flavum hypertrophy causes compression of the cord and roots (Epstein et al., 1977).

The CT appearance in childhood is that of a symmetrically small bony canal with short and thick pedicles (Fig. 7.1). With later development of the bony and soft tissue, hypertrophy of the lamina and inferior facets, the posterior and lateral recesses, appear deeper, giving the spinal canal a trilobar appearance (Sheldon and Leborgne, 1980).

Congenital spinal stenosis involving the entire vertebral column occurs in conditions such as achondroplasia, spondylo-epiphyseal dysplasia, and osteopetrosis. Achondroplasia is the classic example of this group. It is an inherent defect of the enchondral bone formation. In the spine, this defect leads to early fusion of the neurocentral synchondrosis, with ensuing decreased transverse and sagittal diameters of the spinal canal. The gross changes of the spine, with increased lordosis, scalloping of the vertebral bodies, and decreased interpediculate distance are best shown on conventional plain films. The CTMM will reveal the abnormal

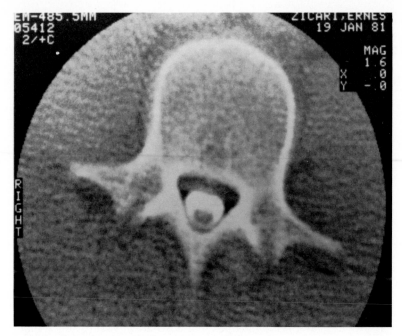

Fig. 7.1. Spinal stenosis. Boy, 13 years, L4. The spinal canal is narrow, and the pedicles are thick. There is a tendency to bulging of the inferior facets medially. There is also a low cord.

configuration of the vertebral bodies, and it will also show the osseous stenosis of the spinal canal, as well as the impingement on the sac and cord caused by the stenosis (Post, 1980) (Fig. 7.2).

Localized Narrowing of the Spinal Canal

Localized narrowing at the C1–C2 level occurs in several different diseases. The reason is most often an underdevelopment of the odontoid process and laxity of the transverse ligaments, as in Down's syndrome, mucopolysaccharidosis, and spondylo-epiphyseal dysplasia. The malalignment of the vertebrae as well as the compression of the cord, is revealed at the CTMM (Post, 1980) (Fig. 7.3).

In mucopolysaccharidosis, as for instance Morquio's disease, there may also occur a posterior slipping of one vertebra at the lower thoracic or more often the upper lumbar region, causing severe compression of the cord (Spranger et al., 1974). There might also be a large bulging disc, causing compression of the sac and cord, as in Maroteaux–Lamy's disease (Harwood-Nash and Fitz, 1976).

Laminectomy and spinal fusion may be performed to reveal the symptoms both of a localized narrowing of the canal and of a more widespread spinal stenosis. However, if this laminectomy is expanded over several levels and the spinal canal is small, there is a risk of herniation of the dural sac and cord through the laminectomy, easily revealed at the CTMM (Fig. 7.4).

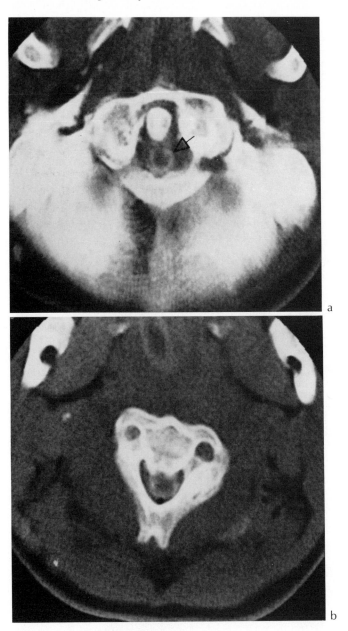

a

b

Fig. 7.2. Achondroplasia. Girl, 11 years.
(a) The odontoid process is high, situated in the narrowed foramen magnum. The cord and dural sac (*arrow*) are posteriorly displaced.
(b) In the cervical region, the anatomy of the vertebral body is deranged, and the pedicles as well as the laminae are thickened, deforming and narrowing the spinal canal.

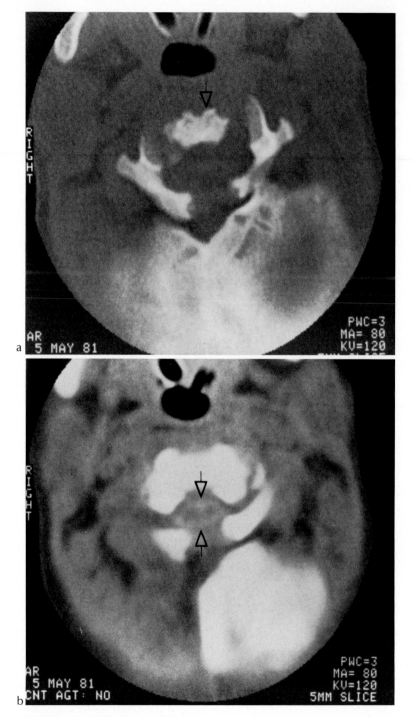

Fig. 7.3. Morquio's disease. Girl, 2 years.
(a) The C1 vertebra has rotated along a transverse axis, and the posterior arch has dislocated into the posterior part of the foramen magnum. Note the defective ossification of the posterior arches of the C1 vertebra as well as of the body of C2 (*arrow*).
(b) 5 mm further down, low window level. The dilated Metrizamide surrounds the narrowed and flattened cord (*arrows*).

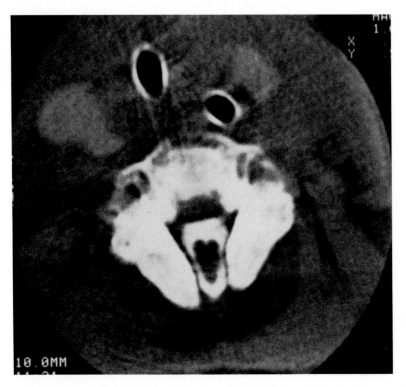

Fig. 7.4. Morquio's disease. Boy, 10 years, C3. Herniation of the dural sac and cord through a laminectomy. The laminectomy had been performed over an extended area in the cervical and thoracic spine. The posterior arches are thick and the ossified part of the vertebral body is small and irregular.

Widened Spinal Canal

A slight widening and posterior scalloping of the vertebral bodies should be regarded as within normal limits. If more pronounced, it might be a manifestation of dysraphism (Chap. 4), and it might be caused by any space-occupying mass lesion within the canal. It is also seen in some musculoskeletal disorders, such as neurofibromatosis (see below), Marfan's disease and Ehlers–Danlos syndrome (Mitchell et al., 1967). We have observed two cases of Marfan's disease in which the posterior scalloping of the vertebral bodies was combined with a widening of the subarachnoid space, revealed at CTMM in early childhood (Fig. 7.5).

Neurofibromatosis

Neurofibromatosis, first described as one entity by Von Recklinghausen (1882), is an inherited autosomal dominant disease of neuroectodermal and mesenchymal origin. The incidence is about 1 in 3000 births (Crowe et al., 1956). The cutaneous

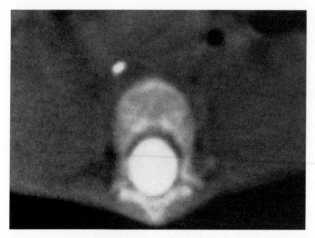

Fig. 7.5. Marfan's disease. Boy, 8 years. At the L4 level, the posterior aspect of the vertebral body is scalloped, and the ectatic dural sac is wide and oval with the large diameter in the AP direction. (In this standard resolution image, the nerve roots are barely visible in the dense Metrizamide.)

changes, including café au lait spots exceeding 1.5 cm in diameter and numbering at least five, together with cutaneous neurofibromas, may be present at birth and usually appear before the age of 2 years. Musculoskeletal defects involving the skull, the spine, and limbs occur in between 20% and 50% of the patients at all ages (Hunt and Pugh, 1961). The neural manifestations of the disease as well as

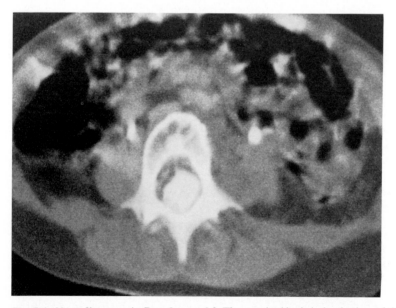

Fig. 7.6. Neurofibromatosis. Boy, 8 years, L3. The vertebral body is dysplastic, and there is a plexiform neurofibroma growing into the anterior part of the spinal canal. The tumor is extradural and compresses the dural sac.

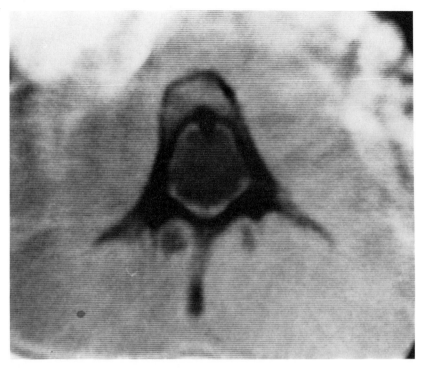

Fig. 7.7. Neurofibromatosis. Boy, 13 years, L4. The lumbar vertebra is severely dysplastic. The dural sac contains Metrizamide and is ectatic.

neoplasms of the CNS usually do not occur until adolescence or early adulthood (Harwood-Nash and Fitz, 1976). The degree of abnormalities varies within a wide range between different patients, from very slight changes to grotesque deformations as described in the classic case of the "Elephant Man" (Treves, 1885, 1923).

The most common lesions seen in the childhood spine are vertebral dysplasias, kyphoscoliosis, and posterior vertebral body scalloping. As mentioned above there is also a dural ectasia often with large dural herniations through widened intervertebral foramina, and there may be multiple plexiform neurofibromas which may degenerate to neurofibrosarcomas (Harwood-Nash and Fitz, 1976). Extraspinal fibromas may extend to the extradural space, being of the dumbbell type with enlarged intervertebral foramina. There might also be multiple intradural neurofibromas without any extradural component (Harwood-Nash and Fitz, 1976).

The CTMM examination reveals the extent and nature of the para- and intraspinal abnormalities (Hammerschlag et al., 1976; Nakagawa et al., 1977) (Figs. 5.3, 7.6, 7.7) as well as the vertebral disorganization (Figs. 7.6, 7.7).

References

Crowe FW, Schule WJ, Neel JV (1956) Multiple neurofibromatosis. Charles C Thomas, Springfield Ill.

Epstein BS, Epstein JA, Jones MD (1977) Lumbar spinal stenosis. Radiol Clin North Am 15: 227–239

Hammerschlag SB, Wolpert SM, Carter BL (1976) Computed tomography of the spinal canal. Radiology 121: 361–367

Harwood-Nash DC, Fitz CR (1976) Neuroradiology in infants and children. CV Mosby, St. Louis

Hunt JC, Pugh DG (1961) Skeletal lesions in neurofibromatosis. Radiology 76: 1–20

Mitchell GE, Lourie H, Berne AS (1967) The various causes of scalloped vertebrae with notes on their pathogenesis. Radiology 89: 67–74

Nakagawa H, Huang YP, Malis LI, Wolf BS (1977) Computed tomography of intraspinal and paraspinal neoplasms. J Comput Assist Tomogr 1: 377–390

Post MJD (1980) Computed tomography of the spine: its values and limitations on a nonhigh resolution scanner. In: Post MJD (ed). Radiographic evaluation of the spine. Masson, New York, pp 186–258

Sheldon JJ, Leborgne JM (1980) Computed tomography of the lumbar vertebral column. In: Post MJD (ed). Radiographic evaluation of the spine. Masson, New York, pp 56–87

Spranger JW, Langer LO, Wiedemann HR (1974) Bone dysplasias. WB Saunders, Philadelphia, pp 143–187

Treves F (1885) A case of congenital deformity. Transact Pathol Soc London 36: 494–498

Treves F (1923) The Elephant Man and other reminiscences. Cassell, London

Verbiest H (1954) A radicular syndrome from developmental narrowing of the lumbar vertebral canal. Bone Joint Surg [Br] 36: 230–237

Verbiest H (1955) Further experiences on the pathological influence of a developmental narrowness of the bony lumbar vertebral canal. J Bone Joint Surg [Br] 37: 576–583

Von Recklinghausen FE (1882) Über die multiplen Fibrome der Haut und ihre Beziehung zu den multiplen Neuromen. A Hirschwald, Berlin

Chapter 8
Scoliosis

Scoliosis and kyphosis, alone or in combination, are important general changes of the spine. They may be congenital in origin, neuromuscular, secondary to other lesions, or idiopathic.

The congenital scoliosis is caused by vertebral skeletal anomalies, such as dysraphism or generalized skeletal dysplasias. The neuromuscular scoliosis may be neuropathic, as for instance in cerebral palsy, or myopathic, as in muscular dystrophy. The secondary scoliosis may be caused by neoplasia, infection and inflammation, trauma, disc herniation, or therapeutic irradiation. The most common scoliosis in childhood is idiopathic. The reason for the condition is unknown, but in some cases it may be inherited, transmitted in a sex-linked pattern with varying expressivity (Cowell et al., 1968).

In congenital scoliosis, as well as in neuromuscular and secondary types of scoliosis, the prognosis is dependent on the underlying abnormalities. In idiopathic scoliosis the prognosis is generally much more favorable, the later in childhood and in adolescence that the abnormality occurs.

Conventional Radiography

Radiologic examination of scoliosis in most cases includes only plain films of the spine, but in some cases a neuroradiologic work-up is necessary: (a) in scoliosis with spinal dysraphism and segmentation anomalies, and (b) in scoliosis with progressive neurologic disturbances (Pettersson et al., 1982). The reason for this is that in congenital scoliosis there might be dysraphic neural changes that should be considered before any orthopedic treatment of the scoliosis is performed (Gillespie et al., 1973) and in, for instance, neurofibromatosis, surgical correction of the scoliosis might be harmful if there is an intraspinal neurofibroma. The neuro-radiologic examination should also rule out other conditions responsible for the scoliosis, such as disc herniation, tumor, or infection.

During the last few years the radiologic work-up in these cases has included plain films combined with tomography of the spine, and MM. However, it might be technically difficult during the myelographic procedure to get the Metrizamide past the curves of the scoliosis and still retain contrast medium concentration sufficient for accurate imaging of the changes.

Computed Tomography

Pettersson et al. (1982) have shown that CTMM may add valuable information to the conventional MM in several cases of scoliosis. This study was a retrospective investigation of 81 consecutive myelographies performed in scoliotic children in our hospital. Of these, 51 children had had a CTMM immediately following the MM.

Out of 30 cases of dysraphism, CTMM added important information to the MM in 13 cases: low tonsils (1 case), syringohydromyelia (2 cases), diastematomyelia (6 cases), atrophic cord (1 case), neurenteric cyst (1 case), and a definite exclusion of pathologic changes in two cases. The reason for the superiority of CTMM was in most cases the technical difficulties mentioned above. Thus, the whole area of interest was not accessible by MM because of too low a contrast medium concentration, while the amount of Metrizamide that had passed the scoliotic curves was sufficient for the CTMM examination. The CTMM also added information in some cases in which the contrast medium concentration in the area of interest was regarded as sufficient for MM.

Out of 12 cases of idiopathic scoliosis with neurologic disturbances, CTMM added important information in 4 cases. In these patients an intraspinal mass lesion was found both with MM and with CTMM, but the CTMM made it possible to differentiate between solid tumor and syringohydromyelia, as described in Chap. 5.

Table 8.1. Radiologic findings at CTMM of 60 cases of scoliosis. Dysraphic changes of the vertebral body and arch are excluded.

Radiologic findings	Type of scoliosis	
	Dysraphism and segmentation anomalies	Idiopathic scoliosis with neurologic disturbances
Normal cord and roots	10	7
Disc and portrusion, nerve root compression		2
Narrowed cord at apex of scoliosis	6	
Tethered cord, thick filum, lipomatous tissue	12	
Myelomeningocele	4	
Diastematomyelia, split cord	10	
Bony spur	4	
Syringohydromyelia	7	1
Large cervical canal, low tonsils	2	
Neurenteric cyst	1	
Tumor		3
Thick nerve roots		1
Atrophic cord	1	

In this investigation it was concluded that in severe scoliosis, in all cases of severe dysraphism, and in all cases of localized neurologic or radiologic abnormalities, CTMM should be added to the conventional examination or should be the only neuroradiologic examination.

Our experience of CTMM in scoliosis now is derived from 60 cases. The changes revealed in different types of scoliosis are shown in Table 8.1 and from this it is clear that most of the changes within the dysraphic state might be found concurrent with scoliosis. These changes have been described in Chap. 4 and will not be repeated here. The tumors causing scoliosis in the nondysraphic spine were astrocytoma and ependymoma with the CT appearance as described in Chap. 5. Also the CTMM appearance of disc herniation, traumatic sequelae, neurofibromatosis, achondroplasia, and Marfan's disease have been described in previous chapters. Radiation therapy, especially if asymmetrically applied to a thoracic or abdominal mass, may cause retardation of the growth of the epiphyseal cartilages on one side, with ensuing scoliosis that might be severe (Harwood-Nash and Fitz, 1976).

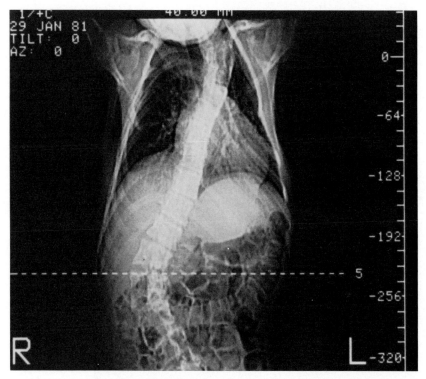

Fig. 8.1. Idiopathic scoliosis. Boy, 17 years. The Scout view shows the degree of scoliosis in the transversal plane. The cursor line denotes the CT section through the upper L3 body, perpendicular to the long axis of the spine, at the apex of the scoliosis.

At the CT examination the Scout view provides information of the degree of the scoliosis in the transversal plane (Fig. 8.1) and from this the gantry may be angled to get sections perpendicular to the spine. The transaxial sections show the degree of axial rotation of the vertebrae (Fig. 8.2), which might be valuable for the orthopedic surgeon (Harwood-Nash and Fitz, 1980). The CTMM also clearly shows the asymmetry of the dural sac and the dislocation and distension of the sac and cord within the scoliotic spinal canal. Thus, the cord tries to take the shortest path through the curves, being situated in the concave part of each curve (Fig. 8.2). The rotation of the cord, following the rotation of the vertebra, is also obvious at the CTMM examination (Fig. 8.3).

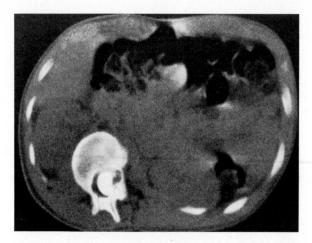

Fig. 8.2. The perpendicular transaxial section outlined in Fig. 8.1. The vertebra is rotated around its axis and its anatomy is slightly deranged. The dural sac and the conus (which is low) are deformed and displaced to the concave side of the scoliotic curve.

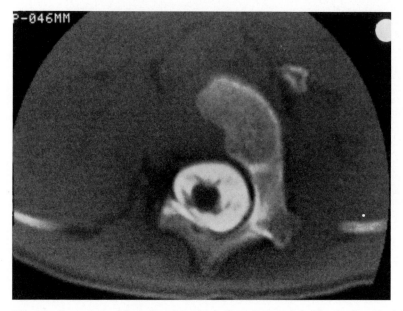

Fig. 8.3. Congenital scoliosis (hemivertebra). Boy, 3 years, L1. The dural sac is deformed, and the conus is displaced and slightly rotated.

References

Cowell HR, Nelson H, MacEwen GD (1968) Familial patterns in idiopathic scoliosis. Exhibit of the American Medical Association, 117th Annual Convention

Gillespie R, Faithfull DK, Roth A, Hall JE (1973) Intraspinal anomalies in congenital scoliosis. Clin Orthop 93: 103–112

Harwood-Nash DC, Fitz CR (1976) Neuroradiology in infants and children. C.V. Mosby, St. Louis

Harwood-Nash DC, Fitz CR (1980) Computed tomography and the pediatric spine: Computed tomographic Metrizamide myelography in children. In: Post MJD (ed). Radiographic evaluation of the spine. Masson, New York, pp 4–33

Pettersson H, Harwood-Nash DC, Fitz CR, Chuang S, Armstrong E (1982) Metrizamide myelography (MM) and computed tomographic Metrizamide myelography (CTMM) in scoliosis—a comparative study. Radiology 142:111–114

Chapter 9
The Diagnostic Accuracy of CTMM

The introduction of Metrizamide and its approval for routine use in myelography has had considerable influence on the present radiographic evaluation of the contents of the spinal canal. During the few years since Di Chiro and Schellinger (1976) first described their experiences with CTMM, the resolution provided by new generations of CT scanners has steadily improved, and the CTMM has now become an established tool in radiologic work-up of spinal lesions.

In adults, it has proved to be of special value in trauma (Post, 1980), but also in several other conditions CTMM may add valuable information to the conventional myelography (Post, 1980; Stokes, 1980). However, it has been stated that in adults CTMM does not replace the standard myelogram, but rather, in selected cases, it acts as a supplement.

To assess the accuracy of CTMM in a pediatric population, and to compare the information provided by MM and CTMM respectively, we reviewed 240 consecutive cases in which both conventional MM and a subsequent secondary CTMM were performed. One hundred and thirty-seven of these cases had surgery, and in one patient autopsy was performed shortly after the radiologic examination. These 138 cases have been reviewed for comparison between the CTMM findings and the changes revealed at operation or autopsy.

Comparison Between Information Provided by MM and CTMM

Below, the 240 cases in which both MM and secondary CTMM were performed are divided into four groups:

Dysraphism (110 cases)
Neoplastic lesions (43 cases)
Trauma, infection, and inflammation (46 cases)
Musculoskeletal dysplasias and miscellaneous lesions (41 cases)

When assessing the results given below, it should be stressed that the CT examination in all cases was a secondary CTMM. This means that the primary MM was evaluated before the CT was performed, and the MM together with the clinical findings acted as guide as to which areas of the spine should be scanned.

Dysraphism

A total of 110 cases of dysraphism were seen. The radiologic findings included in this group are the same as listed in Table 4.1. In *no case* did the MM provide additional important information to the CTMM. However, Table 9.1 lists the 34

Table 9.1. Cases of dysraphism in which CTMM added diagnostic information to MM. Total number of cases of dysraphism in which both MM and CTMM were performed: 110. Total number of cases in which CTMM added information to MM: 34.

Type of information added	No. of cases
Diastematomyelia, bony spur	8
Lipoma—lipomatous tissue	7
Syringohydromyelia	7
Chiari malformation	6
Tethered cord	1
Dermal sinus	2
Neurenteric cyst	2
Cord atrophy	1

cases in which CTMM added diagnostic information to the MM, most of which was of considerable significance. The reason for this superiority of CTMM was in 23 cases that the MM contrast medium was too diluted to give detailed imaging, for instance in cases of diastematomyelia, tethered cord, dermal cyst, and neurenteric cyst. This was most pronounced in the cranial part of the spinal cord, as exemplified by the 6 cases in which low tonsils, consistent with Chiari malformation, were seen in CTMM but not in MM. Moreover, there were 11 cases in which the technical quality of the MM was regarded as sufficient, but in which the CTMM still revealed pathologic changes in addition to those found in MM. Several of these concerned scoliotic patients, as reported by Pettersson et al. (1982). The CTMM also permitted differentiation between solid tumor, syringohydromyelia, and lipoma, as has been described in Chap. 5. In one case, with extradural leak of the major part of the Metrizamide after the needle was withdrawn, assessment of the dural sac and spinal cord was not possible at the MM, while these structures were well assessable at the CTMM.

Neoplastic Lesions

A total of 43 neoplastic lesions (primary or secondary) were seen situated in the paravertebral area or within the spinal canal. Included in this group are cases of neuroblastoma-ganglioneuroma, astrocytoma-glioma, ependymoma, medulloblastoma, Schwannoma, lymphoma, histiocytosis X, and metastases from rhabdomyosarcoma, Ewing sarcoma, undifferentiated sarcoma, ependymoblastoma, retinoblastoma, and leukemic infiltrations.

Table 9.2. Cases of neoplastic lesions in which CTMM added diagnostic information to MM. Total number of cases in which both MM and CTMM were performed: 43. Total number of cases in which CTMM added information to MM: 16.

Type of information added	No. of cases
Extension of intraspinal tumor	3
Composition of intraspinal tumor (cystic/solid)	2
Vertebral lesions (destruction)	4
Extension and composition of para-spinal lesions	6
Infiltration of nerve roots	1

In *no case* did the MM add information to that provided by the CTMM. Table 9.2 gives the 16 cases in which the CTMM added diagnostic information to MM. Most of these cases concerned paraspinal lesions and vertebral lesions in which the CTMM added information on the extension and composition of the lesions. Furthermore, the CTMM showed the cranial extension in 3 cases of intraspinal tumors which was not identifiable at MM, because of the nearly total block of contrast medium passage. However, the small amount of Metrizamide that did pass the virtually obstructed area of the spinal canal was sufficient for CTMM. It was not possible to see infiltration of nerve roots at the MM in one case because of too diluted contrast medium.

Trauma, Infection, and Inflammation

Forty-six cases included fracture and dislocation of vertebrae, cord compression caused by the fracture, disc herniation, spondylolysis, avulsion of the nerve roots, osteomyelitis, discitis, meningitis and arachnoiditis.

In *no case* did the MM add information to the CTMM. Table 9.3 gives the six

Table 9.3. Cases of trauma, infection and inflammation in which CTMM added diagnostic information to MM. Total number of cases in which both MM and CTMM were performed: 46. Total number of cases in which CTMM added information to MM: 6

Type of information added	No. of cases
Vertebral fractures	2
Cord compression	3
Osteomyelitis	1

cases in which the CTMM added diagnostic information. Thus, two cases of vertebral fracture were revealed and in three cases the cord compression caused by the traumatized vertebrae was better demonstrated by CTMM than MM. In one case the full extent and character of an osteomyelitis was obvious only at the CTMM.

Musculoskeletal Dysplasias and Miscellaneous Lesions

Out of a total of 41 cases, there were 13 cases of musculoskeletal dysplasia and neurofibromatosis. The remaining 29 cases included degenerative and demyelinating diseases, spastic or flaccid paresis of unknown origin, and multiple sclerosis. The reason for these examinations was in most cases diffuse neurologic disturbances leading to clinical suspicion of intraspinal neoplasm.

In *no case* did the MM add information to the CTMM. Table 9.4 gives six cases in

Table 9.4. Cases of musculoskeletal dysplasias and miscellaneous lesions, in which CTMM added information to MM. Total number of musculoskeletal dysplasias and miscellaneous lesions in which both MM and CTMM were performed: 41. Total number of cases in which CTMM added information to MM: 6.

Type of information added	No. of cases
Spinal stenosis	2
Cord herniation through laminectomy	1
Cord atrophy	2
Extraspinal neurofibroma	1

which diagnostic information was added by the CTMM. In two cases a spinal stenosis, and in one case cord herniation through a laminectomy, was better accessible at CTMM than at MM. In one case of neurofibromatosis the extraspinal part of the tumor was visible at CTMM, and in two other cases cord atrophy and syringohydromyelia respectively were revealed. In these two cases the contrast medium was too diluted at the MM examination to make assessment of the cord possible.

Appropriate Areas to be Scanned

From the above it is clear that CTMM in all types of lesions may add information to the conventional myelography and that the superiority of the CTMM is most pronounced in dysraphism and neoplastic lesions. However, again it should be stressed that the present investigation is retrospective, and that all the CTMM examinations were secondary. Thus, the area to be scanned had been chosen after evaluation of the findings at the conventional myelography, which in several cases gave a survey of the diseased area not possible to obtain at CTMM. Moreover, in several cases the reason for the CTMM being done was that the MM was regarded as technically insufficient (too dilute contrast medium or extradural injection and/ or leak of contrast medium). In these cases a repeat MM might well have added information to the first performed examination.

It is obvious that if the CTMM had been performed without a preceding Metrizamide myelography, lesions might have been missed because the area in which the lesion was situated would not have been scanned.

However, few, if any, lesions would have been missed at the CTMM if the following guidelines concerning the area to be scanned were followed:

1. *Dysraphism:* The CT sections should completely cover the area with skeletal dysraphic changes, as well as the conus and cervico-occipital junction.

2. *Neoplastic lesions:* The CT sections should cover the area with positive nuclear scan or in which skeletal changes are seen in the plain films, and/or from which clinical neurologic abnormalities may emanate. In cases of neuroblastoma the intraspinal lesions may appear at a distance from the paraspinal tumor, and in these cases a considerable area of the spinal canal must be covered. The same is valid for neurofibromatosis.

3. *Trauma, infection, and inflammation:* The section to be scanned should cover the areas with positive nuclear scan or in which skeletal lesions are seen in plain radiographs, and from which clinical neurologic disturbances emanate. In arachnoiditis the whole spinal canal must be covered, preferably with four or five dispersed CT sections in each part of the spine, using low-dose CT.

4. *Musculoskeletal dysplasias and miscellaneous lesions:* In most of these cases the neurologic disturbances are vague as to the level, and the whole spinal canal must be covered, most suitably with low-dose CT.

As has been discussed in Chapter 2, modern CT equipment is being developed and provides steadily improving technical qualities of the images. With only slightly better resolution provided by the digital radiograph than that obtainable today, the Scout view will be sufficient to replace the conventional myelographic films as a survey of the spinal canal. Primary CTMM will then give all the information today provided by the combination of both MM and CTMM.

Comparison Between Findings at CTMM and at Operation or Autopsy

Of the 240 cases with both conventional MM and secondary CTMM performed, 137 had surgery and in one patient autopsy was performed shortly after the radiologic examination.

Eighty patients with dysraphism had operations, and in 77 of these the CTMM findings were verified. The findings included all types of changes listed in Table 4.1.

In 3 cases there was discrepancy between the CTMM findings and the findings of surgery: in one a split cord was suggested at the CTMM examination, but at surgery the cord appeared normal. In 2 cases the CTMM suggested a lipoma, while at operation in 1 case an ependymal cyst was diagnosed, in the other a dermoid. The difficulty in the differentiation between intramedullary tumors has been discussed in earlier chapters.

Thirty patients with neoplastic lesions were operated on. In 29 cases the

CTMM findings were verified. Histologic examination revealed neuroblastoma-ganglioneuroma, ependymoma, astrocytoma-glioma, lymphoma, neurofibroma, Schwannoma, medulloblastoma, as well as metastases from dysgerminoma, retinoblastoma, rhabdomyosarcoma, and Ewing sarcoma. In all cases the tumor composition (solid-cystic, calcifications, fat) was verified at the operation. One false positive case was seen: a patient who was thought to have an intramedullary mass lesion at the CTMM examination turned out to have a normal cord.

Nineteen patients with trauma, infection, or inflammation had surgery. In 17 the CTMM diagnosis was verified. These cases included fracture and dislocation, spondylolisthesis, cord contusion (swollen cord), osteomyelitis, and arachnoiditis. In 3 cases a normal cord was seen at the CTMM as well as at surgery.

In 2 cases of arachnoiditis there was a false positive CTMM diagnosis: in both these cases an intramedullary mass lesion was suspected but at surgery only changes consistent with arachnoiditis were seen.

Nine cases of musculoskeletal dysplasia and miscellaneous degenerative diseases were operated on. In all cases the CTMM findings were verified. This group includes spinal stenosis and cord compression in achondroplasia and Morquio's disease, wide subarachnoid space in neurofibromatosis and Marfan's disease (autopsy), cord atrophy in a nonspecific degenerative disease, and normal cord in two cases.

As can be seen from the above, the accuracy of CTMM is very high, and no false negative diagnoses were seen in this series of 138 patients. However, there were two cases in which neoplastic mass lesion was mistaken for a lipoma and there were three cases in which CTMM suggested an intramedullary mass lesion, while the surgical exploration revealed that no tumor was present. This demonstrates that the greatest dubiety of the CTMM is in the evaluation of intramedullary mass lesions. As stated in Chap. 5, the differential diagnosis between an intramedullary astrocytoma, ependymoma, dermoid or teratoma, and syringohydromyelia may be difficult. The one case in which a split cord, found at CTMM, could not be found at surgery cannot be explained—possibly there was a discrepancy between the operation level and the level at which a short segment of split cord was radiologically revealed.

Again it should be stressed that the CTMM examinations in all cases were performed after a preliminary conventional myelography, and that the choice of area to be scanned had been made after evaluation of clinical findings and plain radiographs as well as of the findings at the conventional myelography. Thus, the high accuracy of the radiologic examination in the present cases is the result of MM *and* CTMM and the exact impact that a primary CTMM would have had is difficult to assess.

Conclusion

Conventional MM and secondary CTMM together provide a very high diagnostic accuracy in the radiologic work-up of lesions of the spine and the spinal canal in children. The conventional MM might act as a survey which together with the clinical history will provide information of what area of the spinal canal should be scanned. However, in several cases of dysraphism, as well as in trauma and neoplasm, no information should be missed if only primary CTMM is performed, following the above given guidelines concerning the area to be scanned. Moreover, as the technical properties of the CT scanner improve, giving increasing resolution in the digital radiograph, the Scout view may well replace the conventional MM in most cases, and thus a primary CTMM at one and the same examination will provide all information available.

References

Di Chiro G, Schellinger D (1976) Computed tomography of spinal cord after lumbar intrathecal introduction of Metrizamide (computer-assisted myelography). Radiology 120: 101–104

Pettersson H, Harwood-Nash DC, Fitz CR, Chuang S, Armstrong E (1982) Metrizamide myelography (MM) and computed tomographic Metrizamide meylography (CTMM) in scoliosis—a comparative study. Radiology 142:111–114

Post MJD (1980) Computed tomography of the spine: Its values and limitations on a nonhigh resolution scanner. In: Post MJD (ed). Radiographic evaluation of the spine. Masson, New York, pp 186–258

Stokes NA (1980) Metrizamide myelography—conventional and CT imaging. In: Post MJD (ed). Radiographic evaluation of the spine. Masson, New York, pp 537–549

Chapter 10

Adverse Effects of the Examination

The subarachnoid space is a complicated physiologic system, which in the healthy individual provides an appropriate biochemical environment for the CNS, and which also controls the hydrodynamics around the CNS. The CTMM means an introduction of a foreign substance into the subarachnoid space, with ensuing risk of side effects. These may be caused by the needle puncture with subsequent CSF leak or by biochemical reaction to the injected contrast medium. Thus, the adverse effects caused by the CTMM may be considered from two different aspects:

1. General and CNS effects—immediate or late—caused by the lumbar puncture and Metrizamide instillation.
2. Local damage caused by the needle puncture and Metrizamide injection.

General and CNS Effects

Immediate Effects

The physical characteristics of Metrizamide are more similar to those of human CSF and blood than are the characteristics of any other ionic contrast medium. This might explain why Metrizamide has a considerably lower neurotoxicity than other water-soluble contrast media (Almén and Golman, 1979). However, there are several adverse effects of MM reflecting its chemical toxicity. These adverse effects are well documented, especially experimentally and in adults (Almén and Golman, 1979; Baker et al., 1978; Potts et al., 1977; Skalpe, 1977). *Headache,* or irritability in infants and small children, is the most commonly reported side effect, with an incidence in adults of between 21% and 62% of all patients examined. In most examinations, it has not been possible to differentiate between patients getting headache from the lumbar puncture and those getting headache because of the chemotoxicity of the Metrizamide. However, a considerable number of the patients with headache probably represent the post-lumbar-puncture syndrome, as described by Tourtellotte et al. (1964, 1972).

The next common side effect is *nausea,* which most often occurs about 6 h after the injection, reflecting the mean time for peak concentration in the cranial vault (Norman, 1981). Less common side effects include vomiting, dizziness, confusion, disorientation, hallucination, colour sensation, and photophobia. Seizures secondary to MM are unusual provided the patient has no history of seizure disorder.

There are also several reports on the adverse effects in infants and children, but the samples in these reports are very small (Barry et al., 1977; Fitz et al., 1977; Sortland and Hovind, 1977; Strand et al., 1977).

In a recent retrospective investigation, we analyzed the adverse effects in infants, children, and adolescents, to find the circumstances during the procedure that might have an impact on the reaction (Pettersson et al., 1982a). The material consisted of 246 patients; 238 had had a conventional MM, and 85 of these also a CTMM. Eight patients had had primary CTMM alone.

The types of reactions are listed in Table 10.1. Adverse reactions of any type, no

Table 10.1. Adverse reactions to Metrizamide myelography.

Type of reaction	No. of cases
Nausea and vomiting	98
Headache—irritability	53
Fever 38°–39°C	10
Leg and/or back pain	5
Dizziness	4
Rash	2
Diplopia	1
Decreased level of consciousness	1
Seizures	2

matter how minor, occurred in 58% of the material. Of these reactions, the majority (32% of all cases) were mild and of a type and frequency that might be expected from lumbar puncture with CSF leaking (Tourtellotte et al., 1964, 1972). These reactions seemed not to be caused by the Metrizamide injected, or by any other circumstances around the procedure except for the lumbar puncture. The frequency of mild reactions was higher in older children and teenagers, probably reflecting a psychologic phenomenon.

The frequency of *moderate* (17% of all cases) *and pronounced* (8% of all cases) *reactions was directly correlated to the total amount of Metrizamide within each age group and to the cranial extension of the examination* in the spinal canal.

The severe reactions were rare; only four cases were noted (one case of generalized seizures and one of spinal spasms, one of diminished consciousness and one of diplopia). The spinal spasms occurred in a patient who had a large amount of Metrizamide concentrated in a trapped portion of the spinal canal and the other reactions occurred in patients who had large amounts of Metrizamide high in the spinal canal. Otherwise, there was nothing concerning the clinical history or procedure data that differentiated the patients with severe reactions from those with moderate or pronounced reactions.

When considering the dose given to a child, the patient's weight or size is irrelevant. As most of the side effects are a reflection of CNS reaction, the dose of contrast medium given should rather be related to the brain surface area, brain weight, or volume of the subarachnoid space. All these parameters are functions of the age of the child, given normal brain development, and therefore the proper amount of Metrizamide given should be related to the child's age.

In the same investigation (Pettersson et al., 1982a) we found that none of the following parameters had any impact on the severity or frequency of adverse reactions: type of anesthesia (local or general), sedation and seizure prophylaxis, needle size (only 20, 21 and 22 gauge needles were used), puncture site, concentration of the Metrizamide injected, clinical history, or radiologic findings.

The frequency of complications was the same in those patients who had only a conventional MM as in those who also had a CTMM. The patients with only MM had been positioned with head tilted 20° up during and after the examination, while those who had a secondary CTMM were positioned with the head straight on the table during the CT procedure. This change in position did not increase the frequency or severity of adverse effects. Of the eight patients who had only CTMM performed, one had a mild and one had a moderate reaction; the remaining six had no reactions at all. This is in concurrence with the direct correlation between the severity of the reactions and the total amount of contrast medium given, as patients subjected to primary CTMM will get a considerably smaller dose of Metrizamide. This is an obvious advantage of the primary CTMM method.

Late Effects

The development of arachnoiditis in human beings is well known after myelography with previously used water-soluble contrast media, as well as after oily contrast media (Almén and Golman, 1979). Haughton et al. (1977) described arachnoiditis in monkeys after high doses of Metrizamide, but so far there is no positive indication that myelography with Metrizamide in human beings has resulted in arachnoiditis. Nor are other late effects suspected or reported.

Local Damage Caused by Lumbar Puncture and Metrizamide Injection

The needle puncture and Metrizamide injection means an obvious potential hazard for local damage to a normal anatomic structure or to a lesion at the same level as the puncture. This is of special interest in pediatric neuroradiologic cases, as a large number of the lesions examined may be situated in the lower lumbar area, and as the site of the puncture is most often in the lumbar region.

In a recent retrospective investigation (Pettersson et al., 1982b), of 605 patients

Table 10.2. Puncture level and site of Metrizamide injection in 605 myelographies. In 10 cases, Metrizamide was injected at more than one level.

Level	L5	L4	L3	L2	L1	T12	T11	C1
No. of patients	19	181	248	137	9	2	1	18
% of total No. of patients	3	30	40	22	15	0.3	0.2	3

at The Hospital for Sick Children, Toronto, in whom myelography was performed, 587 had a lumbar or lower thoracic puncture, the levels most often being L2–L4. Eighteen patients had a cervical puncture (Table 10.2). The reason for high lumbar or low thoracic puncture was to avoid puncture of large lesions in the lower lumbar area. Of the 605 patients, 407 had a clinical history consistent with a lesion below the normal level of the conus (Table 10.3). Of these, there was a radiologically

Table 10.3. The potential and real risk of puncturing a low-lying lesion at lumbar puncture and the number of cases in which a low-lying lesion was hit by the needle in a pediatric myelographic material. The figures give the number of patients.

Patients examined	605
Clinically possible lesion below normal level of conus	407
Radiologically revealed lesion below normal level of conus	139
Lesion at the same level as the puncture site	71
Lesion punctured	10

revealed lesion below the normal level of the conus in 139. Of these latter, 71 patients had a pathology localized to or including the same level as the needle puncture and contrast medium injection. In 10 of these 71, the needle went into or through the lesion.

Of these 10 patients, 7 had a low cord punctured, in one case with Metrizamide injection into a slightly widened cervical canal. There was one intraspinal meningo-cele punctured and filled with Metrizamide and one syringohydromyeliac sac also filled with Metrizamide. In none of these cases were there any signs or symptoms of adverse effects to the puncture or to the Metrizamide injection. The tenth patient had a Metrizamide injection into a cystic intraspinal dermoid. Immediately following the myelogram he developed paraplegia with urine retention and sensory deficit in the feet. He was placed on steroids and a decompressive laminectomy was performed. He improved somewhat, with increasing strength in the legs and returning bladder function, but still $2\frac{1}{2}$ years after the incident, there was weakness in both legs and decreased sensation in both feet. It is not clear if this damage was related to bleeding after the puncture, to toxic effect of the Metrizamide, or to chemical reaction from the fatty acids contained within the tumor.

In none of the 18 cases in which cervical puncture was performed (using the lateral approach at the C1–C2 level) were there any reactions secondary to the puncture or contrast medium injection.

As can be seen in the above, there was only 1 case out of 605 in which a serious neurologic deficit was caused by the procedure. Obviously, damage to low-lying lesions might be avoided if all punctures are performed at the C1–C2 level, using the lateral approach, or if they are performed as cisterna magna punctures. However, these punctures may also be dangerous or even contraindicated (Cronquist and Brismar, 1977; Gonsette 1977). Moreover, in a pediatric subject, routine puncture at the high cervical level may be still more dangerous than in adults, as among the dysraphic patients there may be previously unknown Chiari malformations with low-lying tonsils. Cervical puncture is also more frightening for the patient, resulting in a higher frequency of general anesthesia.

Therefore, we regard the lumbar puncture, performed carefully, and including an attempt to place the needle laterally in the dural sac (Harwood-Nash and Fitz, 1976) as the routine procedure for myelography, be it conventional MM with secondary CTMM, or a primary CTMM. This lateral positioning of the needle is facilitated by a wide dural sac in most cases of dysraphism.

References

Almén T, Golman K (1979) Pharmacology and toxicology of some intrathecal contrast media. In: Sackett JF, Strother CM (eds) New techniques in myelography. Harper and Row, Hagerstown, pp 7–24

Baker RA, Hillman BJ, McLennan JE, Strand RD, Kaufman SM (1978) Sequelae of Metrizamide myelography in 200 examinations. AJR 130: 499–502

Barry JF, Harwood-Nash DC, Fitz CR, Byrd SE, Boldt DW (1977) Metrizamide in pediatric myelography. Radiology 124: 409–418

Cronquist S, Brismar J (1977) Cervical myelography with Metrizamide. Acta Radiol [Suppl] (Stockh) 355: 110–120

Fitz CR, Harwood-Nash DC, Barry JF, Byrd SE (1977) Pediatric myelography with Metrizamide. Acta Radiol [Suppl] (Stockh) 355: 182–192

Gonsette RE (1977) Cervical myelography with Metrizamide by suboccipital puncture. Acta Radiol [Suppl] (Stockh) 355: 121–126

Harwood-Nash DC, Fitz CR (1976) Neuroradiological techniques and indications in infancy and childhood. In: Kaufman HJ (ed) Progress in pediatric radiology, vol. 5. S. Karger, Basel, pp. 2–85

Haughton VM, Ho KC, Larson SJ, Unger GF, Correa-Paz F (1977) Experimental production of arachnoiditis with water soluble myelographic media. Radiology 123: 681–685

Norman D (1981) Metrizamide myelography. In: Moss AA, Goldberg HI (eds). Interventional radiologic techniques: Computed tomography and ultrasonography. University of California Printing Department, San Francisco, pp 141–146

Pettersson H, Fitz CR, Harwood-Nash DC, Armstrong E, Chuang S (1982a) Adverse reactions to myelography with Metrizamide in infants, children and adolescents. I. General and CNS effects. Acta Radiol [Diagn] (Stockh), in press

Pettersson H, Fitz Cr, Harwood-Nash DC, Chuang S, Armstrong E (1982b). Adverse reactions to myelography with Metrizamide in infants, children and adolescents. II. Local damage caused by the needle puncture and Metrizamide injection. Acta Radiol [Diagn] (Stockh), in press

Potts DG, Gomez DG, Abbott GF (1977). Possible causes of complications of myelography with water soluble contrast medium. Acta Radiol [Suppl] (Stockh) 355: 390–402

Skalpe IO (1977) Adverse effects of water soluble contrast media in myelography, cisternography and ventriculography. Acta Radiol [Suppl] (Stockh) 355: 359–370

Sortland O, Hovind K (1977). Myelography with Metrizamide in children. Acta Radiol [Suppl] (Stockh) 355: 211–220

Strand RD, Baker RA, Rosenbaum AE, Drayer BP (1977) Myelography with Metrizamide in infants and children. Acta Radiol [Suppl] (Stockh) 355: 171–181

Tourtellotte WW, Haerer AF, Heller GL, Somers JE (1964) Post lumbar puncture headaches. Charles C. Thomas, Springfield, Ill.

Tourtellotte WW, Henderson WG, Tucher RP, Gilland O, Walker JE, Kokman E (1972) A randomized, double blind clinical trial comparing the 22 versus the 26 gauge needle in the production of the post-lumbar puncture syndrome in normal individuals. Headache 12: 73–78

Chapter 11
Diagnostic Protocols

The introduction and development of CT and MM has meant a minor revolution in the diagnostic approach toward paravertebral, vertebral, and spinal canal lesions. CT has, in most situations, replaced complex motion tomography and Metrizamide has totally replaced the previously used oil contrast media as well as air in the subarachnoid space.

As has been shown in the previous chapters, the images of the paravertebral structures, the vertebrae themselves, and the structures in the spinal canal obtained by the combination of high resolution CT and Metrizamide are of an esthetically high quality and give detailed and profound information of clinical importance. However, the equipment and its use is expensive and the technique has an inherent risk for adverse reactions and even serious complications. Furthermore, other imaging modalities available, that may or may not be completely suitable, are plain film radiography, conventional myelography, and nuclear scan. These modalities might in some instances give enough information at a lower cost and risk. Thus it is important to evaluate, in each individual patient, the possibilities of the different modalities available, to find the combination of diagnostic techniques that will give adequate information and at the same time minimize cost, risk, and discomfort for the patient.

There is therefore a need for diagnostic protocols, although such protocols can never be more than *rough guidelines* in each individual patient toward the suitable diagnostic approach. In the individual patient, the ultimate choice of diagnostic tools must always be determined by the clinical findings, and the findings during the diagnostic procedure, as well as by the experience and knowledge of the radiologist.

The following protocols have been developed and are now used at our hospital. However, we are convinced that improvement of the technical quality of the CT equipment will further facilitate the diagnostic work-up. As this improvement is probable within the very near future, both present and future protocols are outlined.

Present Protocols

It must again be borne in mind that diagnostic protocols can never be more than rough guidelines for the approach to the diagnostic work-up. At the beginning of a diagnostic procedure, the clinical signs and symptoms and the expected radiologic findings must guide the approach, but the radiologic findings made during the procedure may then alter the subsequent course of diagnostic events. The following protocols are designed to fit most common clinical and diagnostic problems concerning the pediatric spine.

Dysraphism

Plain radiographs (PR) will give an overall survey of the skeletal dysraphic changes. Any neurologic disturbance, no matter how minor, indicates myelography. Conventional myelography will provide a survey of the spinal canal lesions. If there is any doubt of the diagnosis on the conventional myelography, a CT examination should be performed. The CT sections should then at least cover the area with skeletal dysraphic changes, as well as the conus, as a tethered cord might be missed in conventional examination, and it should also cover the cervico-occipital junction, as a Chiari malformation may well be overlooked at a conventional MM.
   Thus, the protocol will be:

   PR → MM → CTMM

Neoplastic Lesions

Plain radiographs may show the morphology of the skeletal changes, and a nuclear scan (NM) should be performed to delineate the area or areas of the spine involved. Conventional myelography might be performed, but in most cases is not necessary. The CTMM reveals not only the intraspinal lesions but also, in great detail, the vertebral and paravertebral neoplasms. If only primary CTMM is performed, the sections should cover the areas from which clinical neurologic disturbances may emanate, as well as areas with positive nuclear scan or skeletal changes at plain films. In cases of neuroblastoma and neurofibromatosis the intraspinal lesion may appear at a considerable distance from the paraspinal mass. In these cases a large area of the spinal canal must be covered, preferably at first with low-dose CT. In cases of suspected CSF-borne metastases to the spinal canal, the whole canal should be covered, again preferably with low-dose scans. If the low-dose CT reveals pathologic changes in a specific area, this might be examined also with scans using higher radiation dose, providing higher diagnostic detail.
   Thus, the protocol will be:

   PR ⟶   NM ⟋(MM)⟍ CTMM

Trauma, Infection, and Inflammation

In these cases, plain radiographs and a nuclear scan will give overall information on the areas involved. Where fractures are concerned, conventional tomography in the sagittal plane may still be useful if detailed reformatting is not possible, while the CT examination has replaced conventional tomography in other planes. If there are any neurologic disturbances, Metrizamide should be injected in the subarachnoid space before the CT examination. In cases of infection and inflammation, a preliminary nuclear scan will better localize the lesions.
   Conventional myelography is seldom necessary, and in the injured patient this

might be difficult, while CTMM is easily and safely performed.

The choice of sections at CTMM should be guided by the clinical findings as well as by the findings at plain film and nuclear scan. In arachnoiditis the whole spine should be covered using low-dose CT, preferably with 4–5 interspersed CT scans in each section of the spine.

Thus the protocol will be:

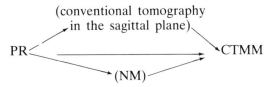

Musculoskeletal Dysplasias and Miscellaneous Lesions

In most of these cases the neurologic disturbances are vague. Plain radiographs of the spine will give overall information on the dysplastic changes. Nuclear scan is seldom of value. Myelography, be it conventional or CTMM, might be indicated in dysplastic cases with severe neurologic disturbances, and in miscellaneous lesions in which surgical treatment is discussed. In these cases, the conventional MM will give overall information on spinal lesions while CTMM may add information on a discrete area with pathology found at the MM or from which clinical disturbances emanate.

The protocol will then be:

PR → MM → CTMM

Future Protocols

As has been stated in the previous chapters, the CT equipment provides steadily improving technical qualities of the images. The information now provided by each high resolution CT section is considerable, while the anatomic detail provided by the Scout view still only gives rough information on the anatomic structures and pathologic lesions. However, with only slightly better spatial resolution provided by the Scout view or any other digital radiograph, we are convinced that the digital radiograph, after Metrizamide instillation in the subarachnoid space, may replace the conventional myelography, giving a detailed survey of lesions within the spinal canal (below named digital myelography, DM). Primary CTMM will then give all the information provided today by the combination of both MM and CTMM. Plain radiography, with its very high spatial resolution, might also be replaced by digital radiography, although probably in the more distant future.

Thus we think that the future protocol for spinal lesions in children will be:

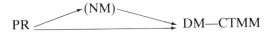

Finally, when the digital radiograph provides sufficient spatial resolution to replace the plain radiograph, the diagnostic work-up for spinal and spinal canal lesions may be done at one and the same examination (except for cases in which nuclear scan is needed). The protocol will then be:

DM—CTMM

It should also be noted that today Metrizamide is the only safe water-soluble CSF contrast medium available but possibly in future protocols there will be other water-soluble contrast media that may be better still. However, the protocols given here, as well as the CT appearance of the pathologic changes described in the previous chapters, will be valid, even if other water-soluble contrast media and other CT machines providing high resolution images are used.

Complete Reference List

Almén T (1969) Contrast agent design. Some aspects on the synthesis of water soluble contrast agents of low osmolality. J Theor Biol 24: 216–226

Almén T, Golman K (1979) Pharmacology and toxicology of some intrathecal contrast media. In: Sackett JF, Strother CM (eds). New techniques in myelography. Harper and Row, Hagerstown, pp 7–24

Amundsen P (1977) Metrizamide in cervical myelography. Acta Radiol [Suppl] (Stockh) 355: 85–97

Anderson RE, Osborn AG (1977) Efficacy of simple sedation for pediatric computed tomography. Radiology 124: 739–740

Armstrong E, Harwood-Nash DC, Fitz CR, Chuang S, Pettersson H, Martin DJ (1982) Computed tomography of the neuroblastoma-ganglioneuroma spectrum in children. AJR, in press

Baker RA, Hillman BJ, McLennan JE, Strand RD, Kaufman SM (1978) Sequelae of Metrizamide myelography in 200 examinations. AJR 130: 499–502

Barry JF, Harwood-Nash DC, Fitz CR, Byrd SE, Boldt DW (1977) Metrizamide in pediatric myelography. Radiology 124: 409–418

Berger PE, Kuhn JP (1978) Computed tomography of tumors of the musculoskeletal system in children. Clinical applications. Radiology 127: 171–175

Bharati RS, Kalyanaraman S (1973) Epidural spinal lymphoma in an infant. J Neurosurg 39: 412–415

Blumenfeld SM (1980) Physical principles of high resolution CT with the General Electric CT/T 8800. In: Post MJD (ed) Radiographic evaluation of the spine. Masson, New York, pp 295–307

Bolande RP (1971) Benignity of neonatal tumors and concept of cancer repression in early life. Am J Dis Child 122: 12–14

Bolivar R, Kohl S, Pickering LK (1978) Vertebral osteomyelitis in children: report of four cases. Pediatrics 62: 549–553

Bonakdarpour A, Levy WM, Aegerter E (1978) Primary and secondary aneurysmal bone cyst: a radiological study of 75 cases. Radiology 126: 75–83

Coin CG (1980) Computed tomography of the spine. In: Post MJD (ed) Radiographic evaluation of the spine. Masson, New York, pp 394–412

Coin CG, Chan YS, Keranen V, Pennink M (1977) Computer assisted myelography in disk disease. J Comput Assist Tomogr 1: 398–404

Coin CG, Keranen VJ, Pennink M, Ahmad WD (1978) Computerized tomography of the spine and its contents. Neuroradiology 16: 271–272

Coin CG, Keranen VJ, Pennink M, Ahmad WD (1979) Evidence of CSF enhancement in the spinal subarachnoid space after intravenous contrast medium administration: is intravenous computer assisted myelography possible? J Comput Assist Tomogr 3: 267–269

Cowell HR, Nelson H, MacEwen GD (1968) Familial patterns in idiopathic scoliosis. Exhibit of the American Medical Association, 117th Annual Convention

Cronquist S, Brismar J (1977) Cervical myelography with Metrizamide. Acta Radiol [Suppl] (Stockh) 355: 110–120

Crowe FW, Schule WJ, Neel JV (1956) Multiple neurofibromatosis. Charles C Thomas, Springfield, Ill.

Dale AJD (1969) Diastematomyelia. Arch Neurol 20: 309–317

Di Chiro G, Schellinger D (1976) Computed tomography of spinal cord after lumbar intrathecal introduction of Metrizamide (computer-assisted myelography). Radiology 120: 101–104

Epstein BS, Epstein JA, Jones MD (1977) Lumbar spinal stenosis. Radiol Clin North Am 15: 227–239

Ethier R, King DG, Melancon D, Bélanger G, Taylor S, Thompson C (1979) Development of high resolution computed tomography of the spinal cord. J Comput Assist Tomogr 3: 433–438

Ethier R, King DG, Melancon D, Bélanger G, Thompson C (1980) Diagnosis of intra and extra-medullary lesions by CT without contrast achieved through modifications applied to the EMI CT 5005 scanner. In: Post MJD (ed). Radiographic evaluation of the spine. Masson, New York, pp 377–393

Fitz CR, Harwood-Nash DC (1975) The tethered conus. AJR 125: 515–523

Fitz CR, Harwood-Nash DC, Barry JF, Byrd SE (1977) Pediatric myelography with Metrizamide. Acta Radiol [Suppl] (Stockh) 355: 182–192

Forbes WSC, Isherwood I (1978) Computed tomography in syringomyelia and the associated Arnold–Chiari Type I malformation. Neuroradiology 15: 73–78

Gardner WJ (1965) Hydrodynamic mechanism of syringomyelia: its relationship to myelocele. J Neurol Neurosurg Psychiatr 28: 247–259

Garrido E, Humphreys RP, Hendrick EB, Hoffman HJ (1978) Lumbar disc disease in children. Neurosurgery 2: 22–26

Geehr RB, Rothman SL, Kier EL (1978) The role of computed tomography in the evaluation of upper cervical spine pathology. Comput Tomogr 2: 79–97

Gillespie R, Faithfull DK, Roth A, Hall JE (1973) Intraspinal anomalies in congenital scoliosis. Clin Orthop 93: 103–112

Gonsette RE (1977) Cervical myelography with Metrizamide by suboccipital puncture. Acta Radiol [Suppl] (Stockh) 355: 121–126

Hammerschlag SB, Wolpert SM, Carter BL (1976) Computed tomography of the spinal canal. Radiology 121: 361–367

Handel S, Grossman R, Sarwar M (1978) Computed tomography in the diagnosis of spinal cord astrocytoma. J Comput Assist Tomogr 2: 226–228

Handel SF, Twiford TW Jr, Reigel DH, Kaufman HH (1979) Posterior lumbar apophyseal fractures. Radiology 130: 629–633

Harwood-Nash DC (1977) Computed tomography of the spine. In: Norman D, Korobkin M, Newton TH (eds). Computed tomography. University of California Press, San Francisco, pp 342–352

Harwood-Nash DC, Fitz CR (1976) Neuroradiology in infants and children. CV Mosby, St. Louis

Harwood-Nash DC, Fitz CR (1976) Neuroradiology techniques and indications in infancy and childhood. In: Kaufman HJ (ed). Progress in pediatric radiology, vol. 5, S. Karger, Basel, pp 2–85

Harwood-Nash DC, Fitz CR (1979) Metrizamide in children. In: Sackett JF, Strother CM (eds). New techniques in myelography. Harper and Row, Hagerstown, pp 139–166

Harwood-Nash DC, Fitz CR (1980) Computed tomography and the pediatric spine: computed tomographic Metrizamide myelography in children. In: Post MJD (ed). Radiographic evaluation of the spine. Masson, New York, pp 4–33

Haughton VM, Ho KC, Larson SJ, Unger GF, Correa-Paz F (1977). Experimental production of arachnoiditis with water soluble myelographic media. Radiology 123: 681–685

Hirschy JC, Leue WM, Berninger WH, Hamilton RH, Abbott GF (1981) CT of the lumbosacral spine: importance of tomographic planes parallel to vertebral end plate. AJR 136: 47–52

Hoffman HJ, Hendrick EB, Humphreys RP (1976) The tethered spinal cord: its protean manifestations, diagnosis and surgical correction. Childs Brain 2: 145–155

Hunt JC, Pugh DG (1961) Skeletal lesions in neurofibromatosis. Radiology 76: 1–20

Isherwood I, Fawcitt RA, Nettle JR, Spencer JW, Pullan BR (1977) Computer tomography of the spine. A preliminary report. In: du Boulay GH, Moseley IF (eds). Computerized axial tomography in clinical practice. Springer-Verlag, Berlin-Heidelberg-New York, pp 322–335

Isherwood I, Fawcitt RA, St. Clair Forbes W, Nettle JR, Pullan BR (1977) Computer tomography of the spinal canal using Metrizamide. Acta Radiol [Suppl] (Stockh) 355: 299–305

James HE, Oliff M (1977) Computed tomography in spinal dysraphism. J Comput Assist Tomogr 1: 391–397

Kaiser MC, Veiga-Pires JA (1981) Sitting position variation of direct longitudino-axial (semi-coronal) mode in CT scanning. ROEFO 134: 97–99

Kaiser MC, Pettersson, H, Harwood-Nash DC, Fitz CR, Chuang S (1981) CT in trauma to the skull base and spine in children. Neuroradiology 22: 27–31

Kaiser MC, Pettersson H, Harwood-Nash DC, Fitz CR, Armstrong E (1981) A direct coronal CT-mode of the spine in infants and children. AJNR 2: 465–466

Kershner MS, Goodman GA, Perlmutter GS (1977) Computed tomography in the diagnosis of an atlas fracture. AJR 128: 688–689

King D, Goodman J, Hawk T, Boles ET, Sayers MP (1975) Dumbbell neuroblastomas in children. Arch Surg 110: 888–891

Koehler PR, Anderson RE, Baxter B (1979) The effect of computed tomography viewer controls on anatomical measurements. Radiology 130: 189–194

Lampe KF, James G, Erbesfield M, Mende TJ, Viamonte M (1970) Cerebrovascular permeability of a water-soluble contrast material, Hypaque (sodium diatrizoate). Experimental study in dogs. Invest Radiol 5: 79–85

Lee BC, Kazam E, Newman AD (1978) Computed tomography of the spine and spinal cord. Radiology 128: 95–102

Lichtenstein BW (1940) "Spinal dysraphism", spina bifida and myelodysplasia. Arch Neurol Psychiatr 44: 792–810

Lindgren E (ed) (1973) Metrizamide Amipaque. A non-ionic water-soluble contrast medium. Experimental and preliminary clinical investigations. Acta Radiol [Suppl] (Stockh) 335

Lindgren E (ed) (1977) Metrizamide Amipaque. The non-ionic water-soluble contrast medium. Further clinical experience in neuroradiology. Acta Radiol [Suppl] (Stockh) 335

Lohkampf F, Clausen C, Schumacher G (1978) CT demonstration of pathologic changes of the spinal cord accompanying spina bifida and diastematomyelia. In: Kaufman HJ (ed). Progress in pediatric radiology vol. 5, No. 11. S. Karger, Basel, pp 200–227

McClennan BL, Becker JA (1971) Cerebrospinal fluid transfer of contrast material at urography. AJR 113: 427–432

McFarland DR, Horwitz H, Saenger EL, Bahr GK (1969) Medulloblastoma—a review of prognosis and survival. Br J Radiol 42: 198–214

McLeod RA, Dahlin DC, Beabout JW (1976) The spectrum of osteoblastoma. AJR 126: 321–335

McRae DL, Standen J (1966) Roentgenologic findings in syringomyelia and hydromyelia. AJR 98: 695–703

Mitchell GE, Lourie H, Berne AS (1967) The various causes of scalloped vertebrae with notes on their pathogenesis. Radiology 89: 67–74

Naidich TP, Pudlowski RM, Moran CJ, Gilula LA, Murphy W, Naidich JB (1979) Computed tomography of spinal fractures In: Thompson RA, Green JR (eds). Advances in neurology 22: 207–253

Nakagawa H, Huang YP, Malis LI, Wolf BS (1977) Computed tomography of intraspinal and paraspinal neoplasms. J Comput Assist Tomogr 1: 377–390

Nakagawa H, Malis LI, Huang YP (1980) Computed tomography of soft tissue masses related to the spinal column. In: Post MJD (ed). Radiographic evaluation of the spine. Masson, New York, pp 320–352

Nordqvist L (1964) The sagittal diameter of the spinal cord and subarachnoid space in different age groups. A roentgenographic post mortem study. Acta Radiol [Suppl] (Stockh) 227

Norman D (1981) Metrizamide myelography. In: Moss AA, Goldberg HI (eds). Interventional radiologic techniques: computed tomography and ultrasonography. University of California Printing Department, San Francisco, pp 141–146

Pettersson H, Fitz CR, Harwood-Nash DC, Chuang S, Armstrong E (1982) Adverse effects to myelography with Metrizamide in infants, children and adolescents. I. General and CNS effects. Acta Radiol [Diagn] (Stockh), in press

Pettersson H, Fitz CR, Harwood-Nash DC, Chuang S, Armstrong E (1982) Adverse effects to myelography with Metrizamide in infants, children and adolescents. II. Local damage caused by the lumbar puncture and contrast medium injection. Acta Radiol [Diagn] (Stockh), in press

Pettersson H, Harwood-Nash DC, Fitz CR, Chuang S, Armstrong E (1982) Metrizamide myelography (MM) and computed tomographic Metrizamide myelography (CTMM) in scoliosis—a comparative study. Radiology 142:111–114

Pettersson H, Harwood-Nash DC, Fitz CR, Chuang S, Armstrong E (1981) Computed tomographic intravenous myelography of the irradiated cord in children. AJNR 2: 581–584

Pettersson H, Harwood-Nash DC, Fitz CR, Chuang S, Armstrong E (1981) The CT appearance of avulsion of the posterior vertebral apophysis: case report. Neuroradiology 21: 145–147

Post MJD (1980) (ed) Radiographic evaluation of the spine. Masson, New York

Post MJD (1980) Computed tomography of the spine: its values and limitations on a nonhigh resolution scanner. In: Post MJD (ed). Radiographic evaluation of the spine. Masson, New York, pp 186–258

Post MJD (1980) CT update: the impact of time, Metrizamide and high resolution on the diagnosis of spinal pathology. In: Post MJD (ed). Radiographic evaluation of the spine. Masson, New York, pp 259–294

Potts DG, Gomez DG, Abbott GF (1977) Possible causes of complications of myelography with water-soluble contrast medium. Acta Radiol [Suppl] (Stockh) 355:390–402

Prakach B (1969) Neuroblastoma and ganglioneuroblastoma causing spinal cord compression. J Oslo City Hospital 19:200–210

Rao CV, Fitz CR, Harwood-Nash DC (1974) Déjerine–Sotta's syndrome in children. AJR 122: 70–74

Reilly BJ (1977) Extracranial computerized tomography in children. Comput Tomogr 1: 257–270

Resjö IM, Harwood-Nash DC, Fitz CR, Chuang S (1978) Computed tomographic Metrizamide myelography in spinal dysraphism in infants and children. J Comput Assist Tomogr 2: 549–558

Resjö IM, Harwood-Nash DC, Fitz CR, Chuang S (1979) Normal cord in infants and children examined with computed tomographic Metrizamide myelography. Radiology 130: 691–696

Resjö IM, Harwood-Nash DC, Fitz CR, Chuang S (1979) CT Metrizamide myelography for intraspinal and paraspinal neoplasms in infants and children. AJR 132: 367–372

Resjö IM, Harwood-Nash DC, Fitz CR, Chuang S (1979) Computed tomographic Metrizamide myelography in syringohydromyelia. Radiology 131: 405–407

Rohrer RH, Sprawls P Jr, Mitler WB Jr, Weens HS (1964) Radiation doses received in myelographic examinations. Radiology 82: 106–112

Sackett JF, Strother CM (1979) (eds) New techniques in myelography. Harper and Row, Hagerstown

Scotti G, Musgrave MA, Harwood-Nash DC, Fitz CR, Chuang S (1980) Diastematomyelia in children: Metrizamide and CT Metrizamide myelography. AJNR 1: 403–410

Seibert CE, Barnes JE, Dreisbach JN, Swanson WB, Heck RJ (1981) Accurate CT measurement of the spinal cord using Metrizamide: physical factors. AJNR 2: 75–78

Sheldon JJ, Leborgne JM (1980) Computed tomography of the lumbar vertebral column. In: Post MJD (ed). Radiographic evaluation of the spine. Masson, New York 56–87

Sheldon JJ, Sersland T, Leborgne J (1977) Computed tomography of the lower lumbar vertebral column. Radiology 124: 113–118

Skalpe 10 (1977) Adverse effects of water-soluble contrast media in myelography, cisternography and ventriculography. Acta Radiol [Suppl] (Stockh) 355: 359–370

Sloof JL, Kernohan JW, MacCarty CS (1964) Primary intramedullary tumors of the spinal cord and filum terminale. WB Saunders, Philadelphia

Sortland O, Hovind K (1977) Myelography with Metrizamide in children. Acta Radiol [Suppl] (Stockh) 355: 211–220

Spranger JW, Langer LO, Wiedemann HR (1974) Bone dysplasias. WB Saunders, Philadelphia, pp 143–187

Stokes NA (1980) Metrizamide myelography—conventional and CT imaging. In: Post MJD (ed). Radiographic evaluation of the spine. Masson, New York, pp 537–549

Strand RD, Baker RA, Rosenbaum AE, Drayer BP (1977) Myelography with metrizamide in infants and children. Acta Radiol [Suppl] (Stockh) 355: 171–181

Svien HJ, Gates EM, Kernohan JW (1949) Spinal subarachnoid implantation associated with ependymoma. Arch Neurol Psychiatr 62: 847–856

Tadmor R, Davis KR, Roberson GH, Chapman PH (1977) The diagnosis of diastematomyelia by computed tomography. Surg Neurol 8: 434–436

Tadmor R, Davis KR, Roberson GH, New PFJ, Taveras JM (1978) Computed tomographic evaluation of traumatic spinal injuries. Radiology 127: 825–827

Tourtellotte WW, Haerer AF, Heller GL, Somers JE (1964) Post lumbar puncture headaches. Charles C Thomas, Springfield Ill

Tourtellotte WW, Henderson WG, Tucher RP, Gilland O, Walker JE, Kokman E (1972) A randomized, double blind clinical trial comparing the 22 versus the 26 gauge needle in the production of the post-lumbar puncture syndrome in normal individuals. Headache 12: 73–78

Traggis DG, Filler RM, Druckman H, Jaffe N, Cassady JR (1977) Prognosis for children with neuroblastoma presenting with paralysis. J Pediatr Surg 12: 419–425

Treves F (1885) A case of congenital deformity. Trans Pathol Soc London 36: 494–498

Treves F (1923) The Elephant Man and other reminiscences. Cassell, London

Ullrich CG, Kieffer SA (1980) Computed tomographic evaluation of the lumbar spine: quantitative aspects and sagittal–coronal reconstruction. In: Post MJD (ed). Radiographic evaluation of the spine. Masson, New York, pp 88–107

Verbiest H (1954) A radicular syndrome from developmental narrowing of the lumbar vertebral canal. J Bone Joint Surg [Br] 36: 230–237

Verbiest H (1955) Further experiences on the pathological influence of a developmental narrowness of the bony lumbar vertebral canal. J. Bone Joint Surg [Br] 37: 576–583

Von Recklinghausen FE (1882) Uber die multiplen Fibrome der Haut und ihre Beziehung zu den multiplen Neuromen. A Hirschwald, Berlin

Weinstein MA, Rothner AD, Duchesneau P, Dohn DF (1975) Computed tomography in diastematomyelia. Radiology 117: 609–611

Wickbom IW, Hanafee W (1963) Soft tissue masses immediately below the foramen magnum. Acta Radiol [Diagn] (Stockh) 1: 647–658

Wilhyde DE, Jane JA, Mullan S (1963) Spinal epidural leukemia. Am J Med 34: 281–287

Wolpert SM, Scott RM, Carter BL (1977) Computed tomography in spinal dysraphism. Surg Neurol 8: 199–206

Young JL, Miller RW (1975) Incidence of malignant tumors in US children. J Pediatr 86: 254–258

Subject Index

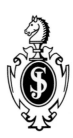

B. J. Cremin, P. Beighton

Bone Dysplasias of Infancy

A Radiological Atlas
Foreword from R. O. Murray
1978. 55 figures in 124 separate illustrations,
4 tables. XIII, 109 pages. ISBN 3-540-08816-4

P. Beighthon, B. J. Cremin

Sclerosing Bone Dysplasias

1980. 62 figures in 218 separate illustrations.
IX, 191 pages. ISBN 3-540-09471-7

A. Wackenheim, E. Babin

The Narrow Lumbar Canal

Radiologic Signs and Surgery
Foreword by L. Jeanmart
1980. 139 figures in 292 separate illustrations,
7 tables. XIII, 170 pages. ISBN 3-540-09443-1

P. Doury, Y. Dirheimer, S. Pattin

Algodystrophy

Diagnosis and Therapy of a Frequent Disease of the
Locomotor Apparatus
With a Foreword by J. Villiaumey
Translated from the French by M. T. Wackenheim
1981. 46 figures. XVI, 165 pages
ISBN 3-540-10624-3

Computerized Tomography –
Brain Metabolism –
Spinal Injuries

Editors: W. Driesen, M. Brock, M. Klinger
1982. 186 figures, 76 tables. Approx. 420 pages
(Advances in Neurosurgery, Volume 10)
ISBN 3-540-11115-8

Brain Abscess and Meningitis/
Subarachnoid Hemorrhage:
Timing Problems

rs: W. Schiefer, M. Klinger, M. Brock
figures, 134 tables. XIX, 519 pages
Neurosurgery, Volume 9)
?9-5

Surgery of Cervical Myelopathy.
Infantile Hydrocephalus:
Long-Term Results

Editors: W. Grote, M. Brock, H.-E. Clar, M. Klinger,
H. E. Nau
1980. 178 figures in 215 separate illustrations,
138 tables. XVII, 456 pages
(Advances in Neurosurgery, Volume 8)
ISBN 3-540-09949-2

G. M. Bedbrook

The Care and Management of
Spinal Cord Injuries

Foreword by R. W. Jackson
1981. 147 figures. XVI, 351 pages
ISBN 3-540-90494-8

H. A. Keim

The Adolescent Spine

With contributions by J. R. Denton, H. M. Dick,
J. G. McMurty, III, D. P. Roye Jr.
2nd edition. 1982. 366 figures. XV, 254 pages
ISBN 3-540-90612-6

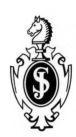

Springer-Verlag
Berlin
Heidelberg
New York

Subject Index

Contrast Media in Radiology

Appraisal and Prospects
First European Workshop – Proceedings –
Lyon 1981
Editor: M. Amiel
With the collaboration of J. F. Moreau
1982. Approx. 139 figures, approx. 75 tables.
Approx. 496 pages. ISBN 3-540-11534-X

Atlas of Pathological Computer Tomography

Volume 1
A. Wackenheim, L. Jeanmart, A. L. Baert
Craniocerebral Computer Tomography
Confrontations with Neuropathology
With the collaboration of numerous experts
1980. 112 figures in 498 separate illustrations.
X, 130 pages. ISBN 3-540-09879-8

G. Salamon, Y. P. Huang
Computed Tomography of the Brain

Atlas of Normal Anatomy
In Cooperation with numerous experts
1980. 226 figures in 359 separate illustrations.
VII, 155 pages. ISBN 3-540-08825-3

Computer Reformations of the Brain and Skull Base

Anatomy and Clinical Application
By R. Unsöld, C. B. Ostertag, J. de Groot,
T. H. Newton
1982. 237 figures including 76 colored plates.
Approx. 250 pages. ISBN 3-540-11544-7
In preparation

W. Lanksch, T. Grumme, E. Kazner
Computed Tomography in Head Injuries

Translated from the German by F. C. Dougherty
1979. 162 figures in 354 separate illustrations,
11 tables. VIII, 141 pages. ISBN 3-540-09634-5

G. B. Bradač, R. Oberson
Angiography in Cerebro-Arterial Occlusive Diseases

Including Computer Tomography and Radio-
nuclide Methods
With a Foreword by A. Wackenheim
1979. 144 figures in 341 separate illustrations.
IX, 228 pages. ISBN 3-540-08898-9

Computerized Tomography

Editors: J. M. Caillé, G. Salamon
1980. 139 figures, 31 tables. XVII, 293 pages
ISBN 3-540-09808-9

J. F. Bonneville, J. L. Dietemann
Radiology of the Sella Turcica

With the collaboration of numerous experts
Illustrations by M. Gaudron
Translation Reviewed by I. Moseley
With a Foreword by J. L. Vezina
Preface by A. Wackenheim
Historical Review by J. Metzger
1981. 370 figures in 693 separate illustrations.
XXII, 262 pages. ISBN 3-540-10319-8

A. Wackenheim
Cheirolumbar Dysostosis

Developmental Brachycheiry and Stenosis of the
Bony Vertebral Lumbar Canal
With the collaboration of E. Babin, P. Bourjat,
E. Bromhorst, R. M. Kipper, R. Luduiczale,
G. Vetter
Translated from the French by M. T. Wackenheim
1980. 39 figures, 85 tables. XII, 102 pages
ISBN 3-540-10371-6

Springer-Verlag
Berlin
Heidelberg
NewYork

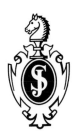

B. J. Cremin, P. Beighton
Bone Dysplasias of Infancy
A Radiological Atlas
Foreword from R. O. Murray
1978. 55 figures in 124 separate illustrations,
4 tables. XIII, 109 pages. ISBN 3-540-08816-4

P. Beighthon, B. J. Cremin
Sclerosing Bone Dysplasias
1980. 62 figures in 218 separate illustrations.
IX, 191 pages. ISBN 3-540-09471-7

A. Wackenheim, E. Babin
The Narrow Lumbar Canal
Radiologic Signs and Surgery
Foreword by L. Jeanmart
1980. 139 figures in 292 separate illustrations,
7 tables. XIII, 170 pages. ISBN 3-540-09443-1

P. Doury, Y. Dirheimer, S. Pattin
Algodystrophy
Diagnosis and Therapy of a Frequent Disease of the
Locomotor Apparatus
With a Foreword by J. Villiaumey
Translated from the French by M. T. Wackenheim
1981. 46 figures. XVI, 165 pages
ISBN 3-540-10624-3

Computerized Tomography –
Brain Metabolism –
Spinal Injuries
Editors: W. Driesen, M. Brock, M. Klinger
1982. 186 figures, 76 tables. Approx. 420 pages
(Advances in Neurosurgery, Volume 10)
ISBN 3-540-11115-8

Brain Abscess and Meningitis/
Subarachnoid Hemorrhage:
Timing Problems
Editors: W. Schiefer, M. Klinger, M. Brock
1981. 219 figures, 134 tables. XIX, 519 pages
(Advances in Neurosurgery, Volume 9)
ISBN 3-540-10539-5

Surgery of Cervical Myelopathy.
Infantile Hydrocephalus:
Long-Term Results
Editors: W. Grote, M. Brock, H.-E. Clar, M. Klinger,
H. E. Nau
1980. 178 figures in 215 separate illustrations,
138 tables. XVII, 456 pages
(Advances in Neurosurgery, Volume 8)
ISBN 3-540-09949-2

G. M. Bedbrook
The Care and Management of
Spinal Cord Injuries
Foreword by R. W. Jackson
1981. 147 figures. XVI, 351 pages
ISBN 3-540-90494-8

H. A. Keim
The Adolescent Spine
With contributions by J. R. Denton, H. M. Dick,
J. G. McMurty, III, D. P. Roye Jr.
2nd edition. 1982. 366 figures. XV, 254 pages
ISBN 3-540-90612-6

Springer-Verlag
Berlin
Heidelberg
New York

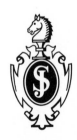